The Essential Guide to Women's Sleep

THE ESSENTIAL GUIDE TO WOMEN'S SLEEP

Supporting Healthy Sleep Practices for Wellbeing and Performance

Dr Sarah Gilchrist

Jessica Kingsley Publishers
London and Philadelphia

First published in Great Britain in 2026 by Jessica Kingsley Publishers
An imprint John Murray Press

1

Copyright © Dr Sarah Gilchrist 2026

Figure 2.2, Figure 2.4, Figure 4.2 source: Shutterstock®.

Front cover image source: Shutterstock®.

A CIP catalogue record for this title is available from the
British Library and the Library of Congress

ISBN 978 1 80501 345 7
eISBN 978 1 80501 346 4

Printed and bound in Great Britain by CPI Group

Jessica Kingsley Publishers' policy is to use papers that are natural,
renewable and recyclable products and made from wood grown in
sustainable forests. The logging and manufacturing processes are expected
to conform to the environmental regulations of the country of origin.

Jessica Kingsley Publishers
Carmelite House
50 Victoria Embankment
London EC4Y 0DZ

www.jkp.com

John Murray Press
Part of Hodder & Stoughton Limited
An Hachette UK Company

The authorised representative in the EEA is Hachette Ireland,
8 Castlecourt Centre, Dublin 15, D15 XTP3, Ireland (email: info@hbgi.ie)

*For my family who provide the sunshine
and inspire me every day.*

*And to those who seek help with their sleep.
May you reconcile your troubled nights.*

Contents

Abbreviations

AAS   Ascending arousal system

ACTH   Adrenocorticotropic hormone

AI   Artificial intelligence

ANS   Autonomic nervous system

ASP   Athlete support personnel

AST   Actual sleep time (hr:mm). The total time spent in sleep according to the epoch-by-epoch sleep–wake categorization

BMI   Body mass index

CBT   Cognitive behavioural therapy

CBT-I   Cognitive behavioural therapy for insomnia

CNS   Central nervous system

CPAP   Continuous positive air pressure

CRH   Corticotropin-releasing hormone

CSA   Central sleep apnoea

DNA   Deoxyribonucleic acid

ECG   Electrocardiogram

EEG   Electroencephalogram

EMG   Electromyogram

EOG   Electrooculogram

ESS   Epworth Sleepiness Scale

FSH   Follicle-stimulating hormone

GH   Growth hormone

GHRH   Growth hormone-releasing hormone

GP   General practitioner

HEFA   Human Fertilisation and Embryology Authority

HPA   Hypothalamic–pituitary–adrenal

HPO   Hypothalamic–pituitary–ovarian

HRT   Hormone replacement therapy

ICSD-3	International Classification of Sleep Disorders – Third Edition
IMS	International Menopause Society
IVF	In vitro fertilization
LH	Luteinizing hormone
MEQ	Morningness–Eveningness Questionnaire
NHS	National Health Service
NREM	Non-rapid eye movement sleep
OCD	Obsessive compulsive disorder
OSA	Obstructive sleep apnoea
PCOS	Polycystic ovary syndrome
PLM	Periodic limb movement
PMS	Premenstrual syndrome
PPD	Postpartum depression
PSG	Polysomnography
PSQI	Pittsburgh Sleep Quality Index
PTSD	Post-traumatic stress disorder
REM	Rapid eye movement sleep
RHT	Retinohypothalamic tract
RLS	Restless leg syndrome
SCN	Suprachiasmatic nucleus
SDB	Sleep-disordered breathing
SE	Sleep efficiency. Ratio of total sleep time to time spent in bed and actual sleep time, expressed as a percentage of time in bed
SWS	Slow-wave sleep
SWSD	Shift work sleep disorder
TIB	Time in bed. The total elapsed time between the 'lights out' and 'got up' times
TSH	Thyroid-stimulating hormone
TST	Total sleep time
TTB	Time to bed
UKAD	UK Anti-Doping
VLPO	Ventrolateral preoptic nucleus
VMS	Vasomotor symptoms
WADA	World Anti-Doping Agency
WASO	Wake after sleep onset. The amount of time an individual spends awake, starting from when they first fall asleep to when they become fully awake and do not attempt to go back to sleep

CHAPTER 1

What Is This Book All About Then?

If you take a look in the wellbeing section of your local bookstore or online bookseller, you will quickly see there are many books about sleep. How to sleep, what sleep is, how to cope with insomnia[1] (a leading sleep disorder), and even books about why we dream and the supposed meaning of our dreams. But what isn't there (and believe me, I've looked!) is a specific book on female sleep and how women have compromised sleep at various stages in their life. In addition to this gap in the market, there are rarely books for health professionals about women's sleep and how practitioners can support female clients or patients[2] at the various points in their life where they may be experiencing sleep challenges.

So here it is. A practitioner's guide to women's sleep. Use it as you need it. Perhaps use it as a guide to dip in and out of occasionally with clients when the need arises, or read sequentially in one go. It's up to you. Perhaps you might need it from a personal point of view throughout life as your or a family member's sleep changes – a useful reference book to help understand sleep at a certain point in life and maybe help empathize with a client.

Some aims of this book are to provide a resource to help practitioners understand and have some insight into sleep health, to provide some practical interventions to help clients attain better sleep and, if necessary, to signpost to the various outlets for help.

---

1   A prolonged sleep issue with symptoms primarily being a persistent difficulty in falling or staying asleep, despite adequate opportunity to do so.

2   A note on clients and/or patients. As a diverse group of health professionals reading this book, you may refer to your clients in different ways. For the purposes of clarity and consistency throughout this book, I will refer to the group of people or individuals whom you support in your professional role as your 'client'. For the context of this book, this can mean a private client or a patient in a clinical setting.

Having a dialogue with your clients around sleep is the very essence of this book. And whilst this book is about women's sleep, this isn't to say that men don't have sleep issues too – far from it. But over the course of a lifetime, there is an overarching difference in men's and women's sleep, and this book is here to explain the whats, the hows and the whys of it.

Another reason for this book is that from working in many multidisciplinary teams of science and medicine practitioners throughout my career in high-performance sport, and latterly public health, I was always surprised at the limited general knowledge and clinical training for all kinds of practitioners in the area of sleep health. Take sleep medicine as an example. This is a wide field that interacts with many specialties of medicine from (and not limited to) general practice to neurology, psychiatry, surgical fields and the more contemporary lifestyle medicine. Despite this, clinical training in sleep medicine is almost entirely non-existent at undergraduate level (Leschziner, 2022a). From a cross-sectional survey of 34 medical degree courses in the United Kingdom (UK), researchers reported that medical schools recorded time spent teaching undergraduates sleep medicine as, on *average*, 3.2 hours. Only two schools had a syllabus or a core module on the topic of sleep (8%) and five (22%) were involved in research of sleep disorders (Romiszewski *et al.*, 2020). Similarly, a worldwide study (Mindell *et al.*, 2011) of medical schools (n=409) reported that, overall, the average amount of time spent on sleep education was just under two and a half hours, with 27 per cent responding that their medical school provides no sleep education. This is compounded by the fact that medical training historically has concentrated on organic pathology to guide medical treatment (K. Hutchings, 2023, personal communication).

In undergraduate medical training, less emphasis is placed on education around wellbeing preventative strategies such as, for example, sleep, nutrition and exercise for chronic disease. Seemingly, it is only when specialisms are selected – for example, respiratory medicine, psychiatry or clinical psychology – that clinicians move into a career focused on sleep. Therefore, some doctors may never be exposed to further training on the importance or effect of sleep health in illness. Consequently, this leaves an area that is not highlighted with patients and leads to concerns about patients reporting that medics disregard sleep-related symptoms and disorders, and medics reporting that they are insufficiently trained to deal with them (Romiszewski *et al.*, 2020).

Equally, allied health professionals, such as physiotherapists or dieticians, also receive very little education on sleep in general training. From my own perspective as an undergraduate and postgraduate exercise physiology student, I can recall only one lecture on sleep in my entire time at university. Only since working with elite sports and furthering my own interest in sleep health, for the benefit of the projects I was leading on and the athletes and coaches I was supporting, did I proactively learn about sleep in far greater detail and its impact on an individual's physical and mental wellbeing.

Having a better understanding of sleep health for medical practitioners, alongside their allied health professionals, will certainly help in terms of offering non-pharmacological treatment tools in areas such as mental health and, more specific to women, the postpartum and menopause transition phases. More on this later in the book.

Where multidisciplinary teams of practitioners work with high-performance athletes, or practitioners work more generally in the health and fitness industry, sleep health needs to be recognized as an important factor in training adherence, injury and illness. Additionally, there can be variable knowledge and differences in how sleep health information is communicated within these spheres. To be able to provide some consistency with regard to the language used around sleep health and some of the practical interventions utilized would add benefit to a practitioner's knowledge base and is a further aim of this book.

This book is not for those professionals looking for a detailed description of sleep or circadian rhythm disorders and associated clinical treatment. For that, I would refer you in the first instance to the fantastic references, the *Oxford Handbook of Sleep Medicine* (Leschziner, 2022) and *The Secret World of Sleep* (2020) by Professor Guy Leschziner, or Professor Colin Espie's useful guide, *Overcoming Insomnia and Sleep Problems: A Self-Help Guide* (2012). Another useful resource would be the International Classification of Sleep Disorders – Third Edition: Highlights and Modifications (American Academy of Sleep Medicine, 2023). The ICSD-3 is the key reference work for sleep specialists for the diagnosis of sleep or circadian rhythm disorders. It follows the basic outline of identifying six major categories that include: insomnia disorders, sleep-related breathing disorders, central disorders of hypersomnolence, circadian rhythm sleep–wake disorders, sleep-related movement disorders and parasomnias. Each of these categories has several subgroups. Whilst some sleep disorders relating to women will be touched on throughout this book, it is beyond the scope of this book to go into detail regarding each specific sleep disorder.

However, it is important to understand what primary sleep disorders are, and these include those sleep disorders not associated with another medical or psychiatric condition. For example, insomnia disorder and obstructive sleep apnoea are two common sleep disorders in the UK (Khoury & Doghramji, 2015; The Sleep Charity, 2024). Of the 60 per cent of the British population reporting poor sleep quality, an estimated one in three people suffer from the sleep disorder insomnia (Woolroom, 2024). This involves a persistent inability to fall asleep or stay asleep, or both, which has been a problem for three or more times a week, for three months or more, and which affects daily living. This is by far the most worldwide common sleep disorder, and it is highly likely that you may know someone experiencing insomnia at any one time, although they may not have had it diagnosed. More on this sleep disorder in Chapter 7.

For clarity, this book is about examining sleep from first principles, what it is, how we sleep and the facts about sleep relating to women, so that clinicians and those working in scientific and medical allied health domains can be better informed to have a dialogue with clients around their sleep health. If, as a practitioner, you can open a dialogue about sleep, this can enhance the support you provide in the areas of, for example, injury rehabilitation and mental health. Similarly, a practitioner working with a woman who is going through pregnancy-related sleep restriction could alter their sessions accordingly, or at least have an appreciation that sleep may be a challenge for their client during that time.

SLEEP IN BRIEF

So what is sleep? Chapter 2 will delve into sleep in more detail, but let's take a brief look at it in terms of what it is and its link to human life.

> Human sleep is fundamental to life. It is a universal experience in that all healthy humans will experience a bout of nocturnal (nighttime) sleep every day. As a species, humans need sleep as much as they need food, water and oxygen; doing without would be fatal. Certainly, with poor sleep a person's daily quality of life is affected in terms of their ability to function, both physically and mentally, and this is an issue we will see women experience on a regular basis throughout their life.

Worldwide, loss of sleep time is at an unprecedented high. As a species, humans now sleep less than ever before. Given the individual nature of sleep, the increasing global evidence of poor sleep quantity and quality, and the link between critical aspects of sleep, cognitive processes and metabolic function, there is now more of a call for governments to lead on poor sleep as a major health risk (Samuels, 2008; Johnston, 2017).

Since the mid-20th century, Gallup[3] have asked people how many hours they sleep each night. In 1942 the poll showed that Americans on average slept seven hours 54 minutes per night. Worryingly, in the present day this average has fallen to six hours 31 minutes and is worsening. In 2023, only 26 per cent of Americans reported getting at least eight hours of nightly sleep (Rausch-Phung & Singh, 2023).

Similar statistics exist in the UK. In their national study involving 8000 adults across the UK, Nuffield Health (2023) reported that people in the UK are getting less than six hours of sleep a night, which is down from just over six hours a night in 2022. Equally concerning is that over half of the UK population do not sleep well, with only 6 per cent of UK residents achieving the recommended seven to nine hours for a healthy adult to promote health and wellbeing and reduce the risk of illness and death (Watson *et al.*, 2015). Therefore, a further motive for writing this book was to help improve the state of people's sleep with regard to increasing their sleep quantity and quality.

---

3   An American multinational analytics and advisory company known for its worldwide public opinion polls.

WOMEN AND SLEEP

A major driving force behind writing this book was to provide a resource for practitioners supporting woman who were living with the pains of poor sleep at whatever point in their lives. This is not to say men don't suffer poor sleep too – of course they do – but for women there are significant points throughout their life where sleep may become a problem. Below is a brief description of some of the difficulties women experience with their sleep, with more detail around such issues being provided in the relevant chapters throughout this book.

On the whole, women have better quality of sleep compared to men. Research has shown women tend to achieve longer sleep times, shorter sleep onset latency (time to get to sleep) and higher sleep efficiency.[4] Yet, in spite of this, women generally tend to have more sleep-related complaints across their lifespan than men (Tandon *et al.*, 2022).

Poor sleep in women is well reported. In 2023, the Sleep Charity, a UK charity focused on improving the nation's sleep, reported that over 70 per cent of calls to their National Sleep Helpline were from women (the Sleep Charity is signposted at the end of this book). A significant number of women report sleep issues later in life, and for most of their lives Mother Nature puts them at risk of poor sleep. In fact, it can be argued that members of the female human species are prone to experience poor sleep through their biology. At a relatively young age, puberty starts, bringing *menstruation* (periods), which can cause sleep issues amid a variety of symptoms such as pain, heavy bleeding or premenstrual syndrome. From then on throughout life, a woman's sleep can be compromised further through major changes in her hormones – for example, during pregnancy and post birth, the menopause transition and an age-related decline in sleep post menopause. More on hormones later as, like sleep, they are a fundamental driver for overall health.

It's not just hormone transitions that compromise a woman's sleep. Women are 40 per cent more likely to suffer from the common sleep disorder insomnia than men (Pacheco & Callender, 2024) and also more likely to experience other sleep disorders such as *restless leg syndrome* (RLS), where uncomfortable sensations in the legs, such as itching, prickling, pulling or crawling create an overwhelming urge to move the legs, and *periodic limb movement* (PLM), which involves repetitive

---

4   Sleep efficiency is a universal marker of sleep duration and sleep quality. It is the ratio of total sleep time to time spent in bed, expressed as a percentage.

jerking, cramping or twitching of their lower limbs during sleep. Rather annoyingly, this can occur every five to 90 seconds for up to an hour (Pacheco & Callender, 2024).

Later in life, women are likely to experience sleep-disordered breathing[5] from conditions such as *sleep apnoea*, an ailment where disordered breathing causes the body to have a lack of oxygen. Consequently, an individual will wake up repeatedly during the night, rarely getting into a deep sleep and therefore experiencing excessive daytime sleepiness. There is more information on this sleep disorder in Chapter 7.

In addition to hormone transitions and sleep disorders, with reference to the workplace, the fastest-growing industry sector in the UK is health and social care, of which women make up the majority of roles. For example, 77 per cent of health and social care occupations, such as nursing and midwifery, are held by women, and many of these positions involve shift work which can also affect sleep (Trades Union Congress, 2018; Francis-Devine & Hutton, 2024).

The hormone transitions, type of employment and sleep disorders can be coupled with the fact that, overall, women tend to take on the brunt of family and domestic tasks, often alongside paid employment, and are also more likely to report pain. A woman's sleep can therefore be challenged throughout her life, and I hope that this book will provide insight, understanding and advice on sleep health matters specific to women. It will start with the challenges of female sleep health by explaining sleep, what it is and how we sleep, followed by explanations of the various sleep challenges women face. I also include many practical strategies to overcome sleep disruption in the various areas of a woman's life and provide signposts and connections to where clinical intervention or other support may be required.

WELLBEING

Before we delve into sleep, and more specifically women's sleep health, in more detail, I should point out here what I mean by wellbeing. The term is often associated with sleep in that it is often said that sleep can help your physical and mental wellbeing. I find 'wellbeing' an overused

---

5   Sleep-disordered breathing is a broad spectrum of sleep-related breathing disorders, including obstructive sleep apnoea (OSA), central sleep apnoea, and sleep-related hypoventilation and hypoxemia.

term; it is highly popular in current times, but how often does one consider its meaning? Throughout this book, I refer to wellbeing as a state of 'thriving' or 'doing well'. By that I mean that a person is consistently and effectively performing at a level which is relative to their life's demands. Essentially, they are productive, fulfilled and thrive and have rigour in daily life. A person who is managing their wellbeing can be said to be coping well with the daily demands of life, however big or small.

I discovered recently, thanks to a colleague in Scandinavia, that the Norwegians have a word that does not have an equivalent in the English language but which nicely sums up the meaning of wellbeing. Their word 'overskudd' literally means having 'vigour' or 'energy' in relation to the demands of daily life, and is a good way to consider how one should feel if achieving regular good sleep. As I hope you will see throughout this book, sleep is crucial to a woman's ability to thrive and, consequently, for her overall wellness.

Equally important to understand is what I mean by *sleep health*, as you will read this term many times throughout this book. Chapter 2 uncovers this much more extensively, but essentially sleep health is a collective term for the various aspects of our sleep that we should consider and protect – for example, our quality and quantity of sleep.

MY SLEEP AWARENESS

Before we dive into some sleep science, I think it is important to scope out how I became interested in sleep and performance as it forms such a large part of my performance consultancy these days and was also the beginnings of this book! Not least, sleep education has absolutely impacted on my ability as a practitioner to support clients with their performance demands, whether it be in sport, industry or daily life. It's also a question I get asked a lot by colleagues as they recognize sleep health isn't an area that is traditionally 'taught' when engaging in academic studies related to medical or allied health professions.

So how does one decide to study sleep when there is a myriad of factors to consider when investigating human health and optimal performance? I first became acutely aware of the importance of sleep for physical and mental performance during my time working as a physiologist in high-performance sport. My role was varied, but essentially involved monitoring and supporting the planning of elite athletes' physical preparation to try to avoid underperformance in training and competition and, ultimately, to perform at their sporting best on an international stage. Training to become a world-class athlete is not a straightforward process and requires years of dedicated hard work in areas such as physical and mental training, and technical and tactical skill development and practice on the part of the athlete and their coach.

The more I investigated sleep and its impact on physical and mental performance, the more I realized the importance of sleep as the human race's largest performance enhancer. This was fuelled by my part in the preparation of the British rowing team for multiple Olympic and Paralympic Games – most notably the London 2012 Olympic and Paralympic Games, where British rowers were incredibly successful.

As a physiologist supporting elite athletes, I was very much focused on their recovery after training sessions and competition. My concern in the preparation phase for the 2012 Olympic and Paralympic Games was that the athletes' external commitments were, if not managed correctly, a potential detriment to training and, ultimately, competition performance. In particular, the ability to recover adequately from training specifically through sleep, was affected by the extra media attention surrounding a 'home games'. Here we had conflicting demands on the athletes' time because they needed to train, but media requests were growing and impacting on their recovery time. Instead of resting adequately after training sessions, some athletes' media commitments were not allowing for sufficient recovery. Combined with a daily commute of nearly 50 miles for some of the rowing team I was supporting meant sleep (and downtime) was potentially being compromised.

This was also a wider issue for athletes involved in other Team GB and Paralympic GB sports. As part of my role with the UK Sports Institute at the time, I was privileged to be in a position to work with colleagues to evolve what we knew about athletic sleep and performance and also how to educate the UK high-performance sport industry on such an important topic.

In generic terms, optimizing recovery from athletic training and performance is essential to allow physiological adaptation. Sleep is the primary opportunity for restorative processes to take place for elite athletes, yet I knew from colleagues' research and seeing it in real life every day that athletes had poorer markers of sleep quality than age- and gender-matched controls (Leeder *et al.*, 2012; Bonnar *et al.*, 2018). Therefore, I started a project to gather data and information about athlete sleep profiles to help with their preparation and recovery management during what was about to become a very busy phase of training and competition, particularly as we got closer to 'Games Time' (the period of time during which the Olympic/Paralympic Games are 'live').

This project idea led to my capturing data on athlete sleep and downtime schedules via wrist-worn sleep and activity monitors. This was one of the first occasions in British sport that normative data on athletic sleep had been objectively recorded on large groups of athletes, with coaches also engaged in educating athletes about their sleep. The fact that British Rowing had a centralized training venue, meaning I was completely immersed in the training environment and had an integral role in supporting the athletes' training journey, had a huge impact on the success of the project. In addition to this was the fact that the then chief coach and chief medical officer were on board with the project and keen to learn more about the relationship between sleep and athletic performance. Without this engagement, it would have been extremely difficult to achieve any kind of data collection or education of the athletes (and coaches) around their sleep health. Previously, sport science support to athletes in the British Rowing programme had been intermittent, and long-term projects were more difficult to administer without dedicated support staff immersed full time in the training environment.

The normative sleep project fuelled my interest in the impact of sleep on performance and became part of my doctorate thesis with my wonderful supervisor Professor Louis Passfield, who sadly passed away very suddenly during my time writing this book. Louis was a hugely positive influence on my practice, doctorate thesis and work since, and I enormously miss having his invaluable knowledge and experience to share ideas with. I also miss his infectious laugh and enthusiasm for life!

Back to the story. Anecdotally, I had observed that where athletes lacked sleep or adequate downtime practices, this often coincided with bouts of illness or injury and subsequent missed training opportunities. This was significant as training availability is a primary determinant of athletic success, and injuries and illnesses represent the greatest obstacle to training participation in athletes (Watson, 2017). As we will see in Chapter 2, sleep is inextricably linked to the immune system. Humans need to sleep to feed a healthy immune system. Elite athletes' immune systems are often challenged due to the heavy training loads placed on them, so combining this with a period of poor sleep means athletes can potentially be more susceptible to picking up infections such as the common cold (Gleeson & Pyne, 2016). This may seem innocuous to the lay person – a cold is annoying, but a few days' rest and all will be well again – but to an elite athlete, a few days of illness means missing a significant amount of training. Or, even worse, a major competition. I know athletes who have become ill in the days preceding an Olympic Games and had to fly home without getting to compete, consequently missing the opportunity to call themselves an Olympian or Paralympian. Absolutely gutting for the athlete, coach and support team, and a hard one to overcome in terms of medal opportunities missed and the potential financial implications of not competing.

Therefore, it's much better to be proactive, and where possible manage aspects of life that can help prevent becoming ill. Of course, one can't control for all eventualities and sometimes, unfortunately, illness will happen, but having good practices to mitigate any chances of illness will help. Maintaining good sleep health is one of these tactics. By prioritizing, protecting, valuing and personalizing sleep (Espie, 2022a), an individual can ensure their sleep is in a better place, rather than being ignorant of its importance for their overall health.

Placing a focus on the sleep and downtime of elite athletes was, at the time of my doctorate thesis, quite novel. Whilst athletes, coaches and their science and medicine support teams had primarily focused on generic aspects of recovery, such as good nutrition, flexibility and mobility, sleep had slipped under the radar in terms of a detailed profile of what athletic sleep might look like. Coupled with this was the fact that in the scientific literature there had been less of a focus on athletic sleep, and those who did investigate it reported loose associations with recovery. As one colleague interviewed for my doctorate thesis about the impact of my evolvement of athletic sleep management stated:

it was pretty clear from my cursory view of the literature that sleep within sports science was neglected, so that there was a gain to be achieved, not just by scientifically linking certain parameters of sleep with actual performance. There was a gain to be achieved simply by formally introducing sleep science into sports science in a way that allowed sleep science to grow in this area, so that if we could foster interest in sleep science, then we cannot only gain immediately, but we could leave a legacy, and there may be something we'd develop from this.

During the time that I raised the issue of measuring and analysing athletes' sleep, I was keen to stress that I wasn't inventing sleep as a new form of recovery! Obviously, I knew it was beneficial to the athletes' physical and mental health, not least in the field of play, but the level of detail in terms of athletic sleep, and the reciprocal relationship between sleep and sport performance, had not *at the time* been investigated in tremendous detail. Added to this, most studies that had been conducted on athletic sleep had focused on international travel and the effects of jet lag on performance (Waterhouse, Reilly & Edwards, 2004; Waterhouse *et al.*, 2007), or used collegiate participants in studies, which did not represent the elite end of the sporting world (Samuels, 2008; Zhao *et al.*, 2012).

During my time of researching athletic sleep, I was fortunate to present some of my findings at one of the pinnacle conferences in my field, the American College of Sports Medicine (ACSM) conference. It was at this conference back in 2013 that I attended a lecture about sleep science and I recall the presenter specifically raising the point that the next big focus in sleep research would be in the area of athletic performance. How right he was! Since that conference, there has been a surge in academic publications on the topic of sleep and athletic performance, and there is now much more available literature and broader knowledge (Gupta, Morgan & Gilchrist, 2016; Sargent *et al.*, 2021; Walsh *et al.*, 2021). For example, we now know that there are three main areas of an athlete's preparation for peak performance that will impact on sleep and vice versa: training, competition and travel (Gupta *et al.*, 2016). There is also much more normative data around athletic sleep, and athletic sleep studies have even developed into the more contemporary esports arena where sleep health is particularly challenged (Lee *et al.*, 2021).

This surge in athletic sleep science data certainly spurred me on to continue with my studies and use the new literature that was produced over the following years. However, studies are still limited in their design, with some inconsistent, unreliable and invalid research methods. A consensus statement in 2021 asked for researchers to better collaborate and utilize more consistent research methods to improve the quality of the evidence and reliably inform practitioners (Walsh *et al.*, 2021).

The good news is that performance-management strategies in 'traditional'[6] structured sports now mostly include a focus on sleep, and as such, there has been a rapid development in sleep-management strategies specifically designed to address the unique needs of athletes in traditional sports, such as rowing, athletics, swimming and cycling. There has been a general move towards intervention 'packages' as opposed to isolated strategies, with many of these intervention packages used within traditional sports, including activities to help with 'load management'[7] and promote sleep health – for example, sleep extension (napping) and sleep education (Bonnar, Lee & Gradisar, 2019; Lee *et al.*, 2021).

It's worth commenting, however, that in the context of female sport, this focus on 'load management' isn't always the case. For example, the experiences of the American women's basketball team were reportedly far from ideal in terms of sleep and recovery post-game, with stories of sleeping in airports when flights were cancelled, thus being denied full access to the conditions and resources that are conducive to sleep. This is particularly problematic given that the men's equivalent basketball team have chartered private flights. This gender-neglected focus on athlete recovery is quite stark given the travel and performance demands of the American women's basketball league, where 12 franchises compete in a compact 34-game season, with teams averaging two games a week (Barnes, 2022). Not least, this potentially could lead to health and safety issues given the proposed links between sleep and injury and illness risk in athletes (Chennaoui *et al.*, 2015; Huang & Ihm, 2021). I have provided more on sleep and injury in the section 'Sleep strategy 6: Physical activity' in Chapter 9.

During my doctorate, I was proud to lead the change in the evolution of sleep analysis and measurement in elite sport within the UK sport system, and following my studies, a further research study through the UK Sports Institute was funded. This focused in more detail on elite athletes' sleep and is a recognition of the importance placed on this area of an athlete's preparation for competition. Quotes below, from

---

6   Sports traditionally involved in Olympic and Paralympics Games such as athletics, cycling and rowing.

7   Load management is a recent popular term for the correct management and administration of training loads (Scamardella, Russo & Napolitano, 2020).

support staff involved in my own research, are testament to the impact that raising the awareness of the need for more athletic sleep focus had. All the quotes are based on feedback during my doctoral research period (2013–2017) and I think it's important to note that the high-performance sporting landscape's focus on the sleep health of elite athletes has hugely developed since then.

So I think the athletes, they do know, and they do want to know about their sleep. But I don't think they really know where to look, or what to listen to and what not to listen to, so there seems to be no guidance or steer from a sport, or within a sport, to say, 'Here's some information on sleep. It's sound, it's evidence-based. Follow this.' Athletes seem to be kind of plucking different platforms of information from out of anywhere, and they're kind of taking that as gospel, and applying that to their day-to-day.

There still wasn't that much going on in that area at the time, even though there was stuff published in peer review journals that was very descriptive, just saying athletes did this, then they went here, then this happened. Which is very valuable, because we didn't even know that much, how sleep changes from environment to environment, and from sport to sport, so I think that's a good place to start. And it is interesting, but I think at the moment it is just that, it is just interesting. It's not necessarily that informative, so the athlete or coach or practitioner can't really do much with that information, other than be aware that their sleep may become something in this environment.

To give an athlete an opportunity, to say that we can actually look at your sleep in a bit more depth, I think that's something that's quite powerful, and athletes buy into it quite readily, because it is very simple, it's not invasive.

So sometimes, doing the monitoring exercise, sometimes that is really good. But sometimes it's what comes after it, just the education of what sleep is, how it works, and what it is not. Those two things combined are really powerful, but which one is more beneficial? I'd say the education side of it initially.

These examples of how I supported the development of sleep health of elite athletes are not to say everyone should be striving for an international sporting gold. Far from it! But the ability of an individual to use their 'energy pot' to their best every day, to consistently perform and thrive in daily life, is significantly affected by the quality and quantity of their sleep. How much or how little sleep an individual regularly achieves will critically impair or enhance their body's physiological and psychological state. So pay attention: sleep health is important!

This is the book I wish I had access to when I was working in the world of high-performance sport, supporting athletes and coaches on a daily basis to consistently deliver quality training sessions and achieve their optimal performance in competition. If I had a resource such as this when first working with athletes and becoming interested in the area of sleep and performance, it would have been invaluable as a means of understanding the basics of sleep and the how and why we sleep as a human species. Also, the intricacies of sleep across a woman's lifespan would have been hugely impactful to my practice, as I worked with female athletes in several sports across my career.

In more recent times, I have moved on from working in elite sport and operate as a performance consultant specializing in sleep health, and now provide sleep health education sessions to a variety of audiences: mainly corporate, but some clinical and sport groups too. Through this work, my other motivation for this book comes from the range of questions I am regularly asked when presenting on a variety of aspects of sleep health. My observations from communicating about sleep health to different audiences and the sleep queries they tend to have are that, overall, people are uninformed about sleep health, particularly how it changes over a lifespan and the basic science behind why we sleep, how we fall asleep and how busy our brains are once we are asleep. Therefore, I will explore throughout this book some of the frequent sleep questions I experience, particularly in relation to women's sleep, and provide some helpful answers to improve knowledge about sleep regulation and health, and awareness of the common sleep issues that people face. I hope this will in turn help you to support clients from a more informed standpoint in relation to sleep. By raising your awareness and education around sleep health, I want to 'unlock' better sleep for many of your clients. Not least, I aim to create an opportunity for you to have a more informed and impactful dialogue with your clients around their sleep health.

Having focused on the recovery of elite athletes during my time as a physiologist in high-performance sport, and now in my role as a sleep health educator, I very much value the impact of sleep on recovery. Recovery in all its forms (physical, psychological, emotional) is a significant aspect of human life whether in elite sport or elsewhere. Human bodies are designed to be *homeostatic*. That is, they need to maintain a balanced state – not too hot or cold, for example – and recovery processes ensure this is so. Sleep forms a significant part of this process, but as I have observed, people tend to not know the importance of prioritizing, personalizing and protecting sleep for optimal recovery. I hope this book will overcome some of the deficits in people's knowledge of sleep and recovery.

I will also draw on my experiences from my time working as a physiologist in high-performance sport, collaborating with some truly excellent science and medicine practitioners, athletes and coaches, and my current role as a sleep health educator, to fill this book with answers to those questions women may have asked about their sleep at various times in their lives: from looking into what sleep is, how it is regulated and how sleep strategies can be used to help women thrive in their day-to-day tasks, to providing information around protecting and managing sleep when women may need the extra time to rest or recover from, for example, menstruation or the often overwhelming symptoms of the menopause.

From a personal perspective, my background in exercise physiology and sleep, alongside my own experiences of sleep deprivation through being a doctoral student with a newborn (hard work!) and now as a working mum, allows me to bring a holistic approach to sleep education, with a certain level of humility and pragmatism too.

Finally, the wider aim of this book is to highlight the public health issue of poor sleep, and to educate policy makers and industry on the importance of addressing inadequate sleep and providing solutions within contemporary society to aid good sleep health.

I hope you enjoy this book, and that it has a positive impact on the way you practise in whatever health profession you belong to. So, let's make a start in understanding the what, why and how of sleep.

Where I have provided advice, facts or figures, these are all based on my own experience or checked for accuracy and relevance. Identified clinical conditions or where individuals have experienced poor sleep for three months or more all require clinical interventions, so seeking advice from a medical practitioner is advised beyond the practical solutions that this book presents. Signposts and referral suggestions are provided at the end of this book.

CHAPTER 2

The What, Why and How of Sleep

This chapter will delve into the science of sleep, what it is, how we fall asleep and why. Fundamentally, it will provide the headlines around human sleep regulation and function. If you're looking for a deep dive into the neurophysiology of sleep, there are some papers referenced and other more clinically focused books signposted.

TIREDNESS

A note on tiredness before I delve deeper into sleep. Sleepiness and tiredness are two different concepts. Sleepiness is a state of increased sleep propensity (likelihood of falling asleep) and is usually described in circumstances or situations where sleep is inappropriate or not desired, such as falling asleep in the workplace. Tiredness, on the other hand, is a subjective experience which is described based on how an individual feels in a certain situation (Grandner *et al.*, 2010b). An individual can feel tiredness but isn't sleepy, a common symptom of insomnia. More information about this can be found in the review on short sleep by Grandner and colleagues (2010b). The focus of this book, however, is women's sleep and manifestations of sleepiness and why these occur throughout the lifespan.

SLEEP HEALTH

I talked briefly in Chapter 1 about sleep health, and a principal aim of this book is to provide an understanding of what good sleep health means and how it changes during significant points throughout a woman's life.

It is a bit of a personal bugbear when people use the term 'sleep hygiene' to describe sleep practices. To me, this term is rather old-fashioned and brings connotations of the cleanliness of one's bed! Generally, the public don't really know what I mean by the term when I mention it and often assume I'm talking about cleaning bed sheets. 'Sleep health', however, is a much more contemporary term and, if nothing else, it is more akin to the present-day health and wellbeing movements we currently hear so much more of. Indulge me a little as I elaborate my standpoint on this.

Sleep hygiene was originally coined as a phrase in the late 19th century by the Russian physician Marie de Manaceine, who used the term in relation to cleanliness. Over time, however, sleep hygiene has become more associated with sleep behaviours and used as a general term relating to all aspects of behaviour or environment that precede sleep. A bibliographic review of sleep hygiene found the most commonly considered components of sleep hygiene were: caffeine (in 51% of studies), alcohol (46%), exercise (46%), sleep timing (45%), light (42%), napping (39%), smoking (38%), noise (37%), temperature (34%), wind-down routine (33%), stress (32%), and stimulus control (32%) (an element of cognitive behavioural therapy for insomnia (CBT-I) training[1]), although the specific details of each component varied (De Pasquale *et al.*, 2024). This is a broad spectrum of topics, all of which fall under the umbrella of sleep health strategies (see Chapter 9).

A leading pioneer of sleep, Peter Hauri, famously didn't like the term 'sleep hygiene', but used it 'for lack of a better term', and unfortunately it stuck! He described sleep hygiene as being:

> intended to provide information about lifestyle (diet, exercise, substance use) and environmental factors (light, noise, temperature) that may interfere with or promote better sleep. Sleep hygiene also may include general sleep facilitating recommendations, such as allowing enough time to relax before bedtime, and information about the benefits of maintaining a regular sleep schedule. (Hauri, 1977)

I accept that 'sleep hygiene' is a commonly used term among clinicians, but whilst this is a small point on semantics, I prefer the term 'sleep

---

1   CBT-I is a form of cognitive therapy used to treat insomnia. More detail on CBT-I is provided throughout this book.

health'. From the many presentations I have given to various audiences, I have found that, for many people, sleep health terminology resonates with the fact that I am advising on an aspect of health that impacts on the rest of their immune, metabolic, cardiovascular, cognitive and behavioural health (Grandner *et al.*, 2010a; Grandner, 2022). Once audiences understand that sleep health is a generic term for the fundamental aspects of good sleep, outlined below, this aids their understanding of how to work towards achieving consistently good sleep.

It's important to note that practical sleep health strategies (traditionally referred to as 'sleep hygiene practices') aren't meant as standalone interventions for sleep disorders. Where clinical input is required, clients should be referred as appropriate.

So, what do I mean by sleep health? Really, it is a generic term for the various aspects of sleep that people should consider and protect. The American Academy of Sleep Medicine position statement on sleep health (2015) describes it as a 'collective state requiring adequate sleep duration, appropriate timing, regularity, the absence of sleep disorders, and good quality'. Therefore, sleep health is multidimensional. Figure 2.1 illustrates the various aspects of sleep health along with some example questions you may ask your clients if discussing their sleep health.

Sleep health variables can be measured subjectively through self-reporting questionnaires, or objectively through the various sleep technology devices available (Ramar *et al.*, 2021). More on this later in this chapter, but initially let's look at the various aspects of sleep health.

Take sleep duration first, otherwise referred to as sleep quantity. Typically, a healthy adult requires, *on average*, seven to nine hours of good-quality sleep per night to reduce morbidity and mortality risks (Chennaoui *et al.*, 2015). There are exceptions to this, and it is widely recognized that sleep duration is a highly individualized requirement which is influenced by genetic, behavioural, medical and environmental factors. Table 2.1 shows the different sleep duration recommendations over the course of a lifespan and the buffer zone for each age group where sleep duration may be appropriate. Outside of these areas are the 'no go' areas where the amount of sleep isn't recommended for that age group. For example, a healthy young adult is recommended to have between seven and nine hours' sleep (give or take), but it is not recommended that they regularly have less than seven or more than 11 hours of sleep.

Adequate sleep duration
How much did you sleep over 24 hours?

When do you sleep?

Quantity

Appropriate timing

Regularity

Healthy sleep

Absence of sleep disorder

Do you have consistent
sleep and wake times?

Good quality

Alertness

How well do you fall asleep and stay
asleep? (efficiency)

Do you maintain good focus and
attention during waking hours?

Do you feel satisfied with your sleep?

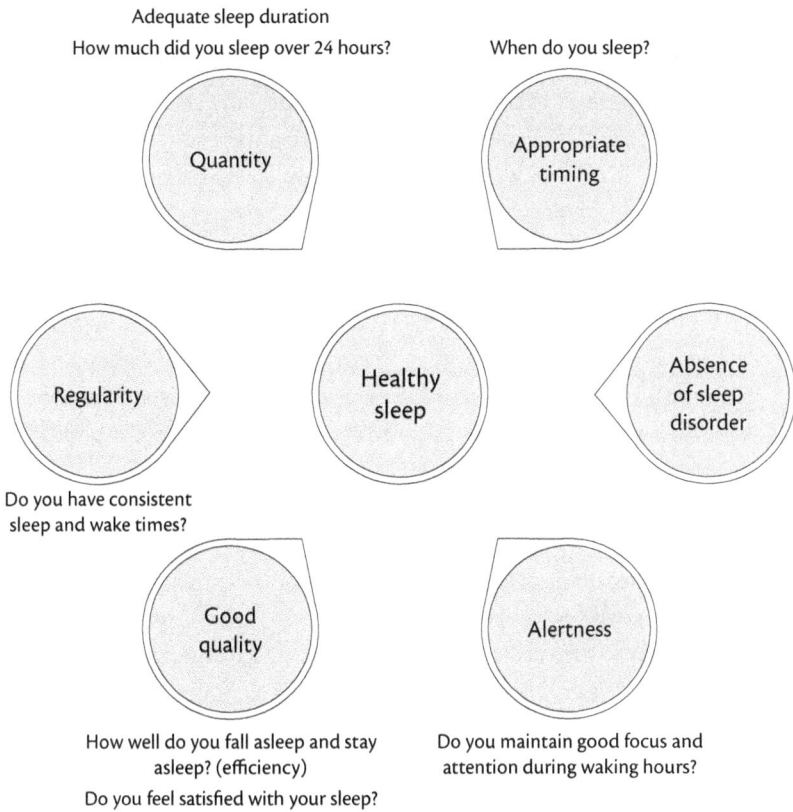

FIGURE 2.1 COMPONENTS OF SLEEP HEALTH

Table 2.1 Sleep duration recommendations (hours) (adapted from Rausch-Phung & Singh, 2023)

	Maybe appropriate	Recommended	Maybe appropriate
Newborn	11–13	14–17 (including naps)	18–19
Infant	10–11	12–15 (including naps)	16–18
Toddler	9–10	11–14 (including naps)	15–16
Preschool	8–9	10–13 (including naps)	14
School age	7–8	9–11	12
Teen	7	8–10	11
Young adult	6	7–9	10–11
Adult	6	7–9	10
Older adult	5–6	7–8	9

If you're looking to advise clients on their sleep duration, then a simple and useful method to ascertain if a healthy adult is getting enough sleep, or to subjectively measure their sleep quantity requirements, is to assess how they feel on waking. Most people will feel a bit groggy in the morning, but if, on the whole, an individual feels recovered and satisfied following a bout of nighttime sleep and is generally alert, refreshed and fully productive during a working day, then the chances are they are getting enough sleep. If they are falling asleep before lunch, have excess daytime sleepiness or are having an inordinate amount of caffeine to maintain alertness, then perhaps they need to look at the amount of sleep they're getting. The practical strategies presented in Chapter 9 should help with this.

A validated questionnaire that is also useful to subjectively assess a client's sleep is the Epworth Sleepiness Scale (Johns, 1990). This is a commonly used subjective, single-answer questionnaire focusing on daytime sleepiness and is widely available online (signposted at the end of this book). It is often regarded as the easiest and most commonly used measure for clinicians and researchers to measure daytime sleepiness (Lapin *et al.*, 2018).

I am always wary of attaching a number to sleep quantity as I find people get hung up on the number, rather than assessing how content they feel on a daily basis in relation to their sleep. For example, are they satisfied with their sleep bout in terms of how alert they feel the following day? There are guidelines for sleep quantity which do serve a purpose, but encouraging people to focus on getting a good regular opportunity to sleep and how adequate they feel after their sleep bout is, in my opinion, better than advising on a specific number of hours of sleep. Not least, a person's desired sleep quantity will undoubtedly change as their life demands fluctuate and they age.

Regarding appropriate *timings* for sleep health, I would advise individuals that they should be getting to bed and getting up at times to suit their lifestyle and daily time commitments. With this comes *regularity* in the sense that individuals need a consistent bout of nocturnal sleep within the 24-hour earthly spin and that it should be, ideally, at the same time of day. The section 'Circadian rhythms' later in this chapter highlights the importance of regularity in our sleep schedules and their timing, along with the scientific rationale for consistent sleep schedules. Do advise your clients to be pragmatic, though. Sometimes life gets in the way, such as work pressures or illness. However, on the whole an individual should be aiming for a regular sleep schedule over the course of a normal week. Obviously, this depends on a person's circumstances – for example, they may work shifts – but nonetheless, *where possible*, having a good routine of overnight sleep is vitally important to overall health.

This regular bout of sleep should also be of sufficient quality. Whilst the recommended seven to nine hours of sleep for a healthy adult is good, this has to encompass all aspects of sleep architecture – for example, deep and light sleep (more on this later in this chapter) – in order for full restoration of physical and mental processes.

Historically, sleep quality has been described as a complex phenomenon, hard to define and measure objectively (Buysse *et al.*, 1989). It typically focuses on issues initiating or maintaining sleep or early morning awakening (Gupta *et al.*, 2016) and is associated with better health, a reduction in daytime sleepiness and greater overall feelings of wellbeing and cognitive functioning (Hyyppa & Kronholm, 1989). Sleep quality is therefore related to a person's satisfaction with their sleep experience, involving aspects of sleep initiation, sleep maintenance, sleep quantity and how refreshed they feel upon wakening (Kline, 2020; Wang *et al.*, 2020). The National Sleep Foundation listed key indicators of good sleep quality as being an increase in sleeping time whilst in bed (at least 85% of the total time), falling asleep in 30 minutes or less, waking up no more than once per night, and being awake for 20 minutes or less after initially falling asleep (Ohayon *et al.*, 2017).

However, it's important to note that the odd bad night's sleep won't be too much of an issue and can be overcome relatively easily with, for example, some light exercise, hydration and fresh air. However, from a health and safety point of view, cognitive abilities are diminished, so activities such as operating machinery and driving are not advised. Typically, after about 16 hours of no sleep the human body starts to feel the impact of this sleep restriction, and certainly any longer than that and a person would be cognitively similar to someone who is over the legal limit of alcohol to drive. An individual enters a significantly sleep-restricted state after successive nights of poor sleep, and this is where physical and mental issues arise.

A note on sleep terminology here. Sleep restriction occurs when an individual falls asleep later or wakes earlier than normal; that is, their normal sleep–wake cycle is *partially* disturbed. Chronic sleep restriction is frequently experienced due to medical conditions, sleep disorders, work demands, social and domestic responsibilities, and lifestyle. Restricted sleep, which occurs when someone routinely gets significantly less sleep than they need, is one of the most common reasons that adults experience sleep loss. Some examples where individuals experience sleep restriction are through shift work, late-night studying or being a new parent. During these circumstances, an individual will get some sleep on the whole, but daily function, such as cognition, is compromised somewhat (Banks & Dinges, 2007; Fullagar *et al.*, 2015).

Sleep restriction over time results in a form of sleep debt or 'social jet lag', which does need to be managed, but it is not as devastating as clinical sleep deprivation such as from insomnia. Social jet lag is essentially a misalignment between the timing of a person's demands of work, school, life and so on and their natural innate circadian rhythm. A good example would be where an individual works late and gets up early in the week and then sleeps longer at the weekend as they suffer a 'sleep hangover' from the shorter sleep they've experienced in the week and the resultant misaligned circadian rhythm. Regarding sleep health, this is where sleep quality suffers. Poor sleep quality, or insufficient sleep – for example, regularly achieving less than seven hours – is considered a public health concern and has been identified as a risk factor for several critical health issues such as immune system dysfunction, type 2 diabetes, mental health disorders and ultimately an overall increased risk of death (Schwartz & Roth, 2008; Besedovsky, Lange & Born, 2012; Xie *et al.*, 2013; American Academy of Sleep Medicine, 2015; Watson *et al.*, 2015; Nunn, Samson & Krystal, 2016).

At the other end of the sleep debt continuum is sleep deprivation. This generally refers to extreme cases of sleep loss, whereby an individual does not sleep at all for a *prolonged* period (i.e. whole nights). Sleep deprivation is very serious and, in general terms, is a huge problem as it induces sleepiness, often excessive, and reduces daytime alertness and performance (Leger *et al.*, 2008).

Finally, the concept of sleep health also includes an absence of a sleep or circadian rhythm disorder.

More on these later in relation to female sleep, but suffice to say, in general, there is a higher prevalence of sleep disorders (e.g. insomnia or restless leg syndrome, particularly in later life) and dissatisfaction with sleep in women (Nowakowski, Meers & Heimbach, 2013). As I've

mentioned previously, that's not to say men don't suffer sleep or circadian rhythm disorders, but this is not the focus of this book.

More specifically, sleep health can be broken down into the impact it
has on all aspects of our health. From an individual, social and societal
level, sleep health impacts our metabolic, cardiovascular, immunolog-
ical, behavioural and cognitive health (Grandner *et al.*, 2010a; Grandner, 2022). If we sleep poorly, we are affected in terms of our emotions,
behaviour, cognitive function and ability to fight off infection. This has
a known effect for humans socially and, on a much wider scale, on society in terms of productivity lost in the workplace and the cost to public
health to help society to be well again. Chapter 10 has more information
on productivity in the workplace in relation to sleep, where you will
learn of the staggering annual economic cost to UK industry due to
sleep-related issues.

Considering the term 'sleep health', how much time do your clients
pay attention to theirs? I'm always struck by the fact that sleep makes
people feel so much better compared to the alternative sleep-restricted
state, yet, as a species, humans are generally not very good at addressing good sleep health. Having a strategy to achieve good sleep is paramount in improving sleep health, yet how many individuals consider
their sleep and pay attention to it and how it makes them feel if they've
had enough or not enough? How many people actively devise a strategy
or intervention to allow them to consistently hit the pillow each night
at a regular time, with the specific prerequisites to their sleep onset
addressed? From delivering many sleep health education sessions to a
variety of audiences, I would argue that not many people address their
sleep to the extent they perhaps should. I hope that this book will help
tackle this by educating readers on sleep health and, in turn, help practitioners to have a dialogue about sleep with their clients.

To help the cause of considering sleep health, Professor Colin Espie
from the University of Oxford Nuffield Department of Clinical Neu-
rosciences described five principles of good sleep health, which are
outlined in Table 2.2. You can find a detailed description of each principle in Professor Espie's 2022 paper (Espie 2022a). I particularly like
the idea of these five principles and advocate them many times in my
sleep education sessions as they perfectly encapsulate what a strategy

for good sleep health should involve. They are relatively simple to live by and, if used regularly, will help improve overall sleep health on an individual and societal level in a relatively short space of time. However, if an individual has long-term sleep restriction, circadian rhythm misalignment or an untreated sleep disorder, they should be referred for specialist guidance; comprehensive signposting for sleep referral and help is provided at the end of this book.

Table 2.2 Principles of good sleep (Espie, 2022a)

1.	**Value** sleep as something crucial to life, and take it seriously
2.	**Prioritize** sleep by putting sleep first when making choices about what one wants to do
3.	**Personalize** sleep by finding the 'sleep window' that works best for the individual
4.	**Trust** that sleep is a natural process and that sleep will get itself into a good pattern
5.	**Protect** sleep by avoiding or preventing things that can upset it

The other caveat to these principles of good sleep health is to remind your clients to be pragmatic when considering their sleep health and attempting to abide by these principles. As I've said already, sometimes life gets in the way, so you can't be idealistic about sleep; that's when sleep issues can potentially occur. If, on the whole, an individual is protecting and personalizing their sleep window and prioritizing and valuing their sleep, then they are in a better place than being ignorant of these facts.

THE IMPACT OF GOOD SLEEP

Referring back to my previous role in high-performance sport, we would focus on determinants of performance a lot. For example, what are the physical, technical, tactical and psychological determinants of a certain sport or event that will enable an athlete to win a gold medal? In order to achieve these determinants, a vast array of factors need to be considered, not least talent and genetics, before any type of training is imposed. Yet sleep, I would argue, is the biggest impact factor on any determinant of performance. If an athlete doesn't sleep well, they won't train well or learn well, nor be technically and tactically proficient in their chosen sport. My work in sport therefore led me to be an advocate of the fact that sleep is the biggest performance enhancer. It's free and readily available if a person trusts the natural process of sleep and protects and prioritizes their sleep time. Valuing sleep as an important part of a working week and personalizing a sleep window will go a long way in improving people's short- and long-term physical and mental health and wellbeing.

The good news is that people can address their sleep health relatively easily and, if struggling with it, can make some pretty straightforward changes to achieve a marked gain in their sleep quality and quantity (in the absence of a sleep disorder). I am often asked what single piece of advice I would offer regarding sleep, and put simply, it is to consider having a strategy for good sleep health. Pay attention to sleep. Have the opportunity to regularly get good sleep quality and quantity. Follow the five principles outlined above and regularly check in on one's sleep in relation to how general life and work 'performance' are going.

So, without further ado, let's look into sleep, starting off with the mystery of what it actually is.

WHAT IS SLEEP?

Sleep has been studied in detail since the early 20th century (Piéron, 1913). It is researched in many scientific and medical domains, including physiology, psychology and cardio-respiratory medicine (Xie *et al.*, 2013; Nunn *et al.*, 2016), which makes it multidisciplinary in its nature and highlights its complexity. The fact that no scientific or medical specialism independently 'owns sleep' not only emphasizes the intricacy of sleep, but also makes it all the more intriguing as a biological process.

Since the mid-2000s sleep research has exploded, with increases in the publication of original science on sleep in high-impact general science and medical journals such as *The Lancet* and *Nature*. This international growth of original sleep science provides a marvellous opportunity for researchers to communicate the value of their discoveries of the mechanisms and functions of sleep and its contribution to health, safety and, ultimately, quality of life (Dinges, 2014).

Until fairly recently, sleep was seen as a bit of a biological mystery. Whilst much was known about the human body and its biological functioning, the exact mechanisms for sleep, its true function and the reason the human species needs it and with such regularity had remained somewhat unknown. Whilst this knowledge gap has narrowed in recent years, some sleep mysteries still remain. Why, for example, do adult humans need to sleep for approximately seven to nine hours within every 24-hour cycle? Why not sleep another way? Dolphins, for example, swim along in the ocean with half their brain asleep and half awake. This is called unihemispheric sleep, a technique thought to have evolved to allow dolphins to breathe at the surface of water and be aware of predators even when snoozing. This ability to shut down half of a brain might be quite appealing for a person with a lot to do. It seems quite an efficient way of dealing with life's demands if one could get some of the 'to do' list ticked off whilst half the brain sleeps. However, humans aren't built that way and suffer dramatically if they have chronic restricted sleep. It is an important and insistent basic physiological function.

What is known about sleep is that it supports life. It is universal in that everyone sleeps to a greater or lesser extent. It is reversable in the sense that individuals naturally awake following a bout of sleep, which is different to other states of unconsciousness, such as a coma or anaesthesia. Sleep must be important to humans because, as a species, evolution has conserved the sleep state, albeit in a shortened version – humans now tend to sleep for less long than ever before. However, how much of an individual's time spent asleep is evolutionary or a result of industrialization, contemporary work cultures and the 'Generation Z'[2] technology revolution is open for debate. More on this in Chapter 10.

Notable researchers in sleep, Borbély et al. (2016) stated that sleep must 'subserve long term maintenance of cerebral integrity', meaning that sleep serves to maintain brain function. It is the plasticity of the brain (the ability to create and adapt neuronal pathways) that causes the demand for sleep in that the synaptic and cellular processes that have been challenged during the waking state are re-established during sleep. Sleep therefore is a period of restorative responsiveness in which the dynamic processes managing it intrinsically interact (Morgan, 2016; Morgan, personal communication, 2016).

---

2   Generation Z is the demographic cohort succeeding Millennials (born 1981–1996) and preceding Generation Alpha (born 2010s to mid-2020s). Generation Z are people born in the mid to late 1990s through to the early 2010s.

In essence, sleep is a primal need, considered critical to human physiological and cognitive function (Fullagar *et al.*, 2015); without it, we would perish. It is a reoccurring habitual event of intervals throughout a 24-hour period and involves an individual being in a state of reduced movement and sensory responsiveness. It is more likely that it has a multipurpose role for restorative, neuro-metabolic and cognitive benefits than a single biological purpose (Frank & Benington, 2006).

Sleep doesn't just serve to prevent daytime sleepiness; it offers respite and recuperation from the physical and mental demands of being awake and prepares the body for the next wake-related energy burst. It is also fundamental to conserving energy stores and directing them to important biological processes such as metabolism, energy conservation, physical growth and development, the renewal and repair of body tissues and muscle restoration (Takahashi *et al.*, 1968; Schwartz and Roth, 2008; Besedovsky *et al.*, 2012; Xie *et al.*, 2013). By helping humans save energy, in evolutionary terms, they can use more energy for wake-related features such as awareness, hunting for food and reproduction. Sleep also plays a central role in many psycho-physiological processes, such as behaviour, and is inextricably linked to an individual's ability to fight infection (immune system maintenance). Cognition function, memory consolidation and ability to regulate emotions are all also related to sleep (Samuels, 2008; Myllymäki *et al.* 2011; Venter, 2012). Wow, what a list!

Because individuals vary in their need for sleep, it can be easy to underestimate the value of sleep, yet it is a fundamental daily function which all human beings require. Certainly, without sleep, a human will eventually die. Whilst it's not clear how long humans can last without sleep, significant symptoms are present within 36 hours of having no sleep. Immune function is certainly compromised, along with profound limitations in cognition – that is, the ability to think, multitask, remember details and pay attention. The longest recorded period a human has gone without sleep was set in 1964 by an American, Randy Gardner, who, aged 17 years old, stayed awake for *eleven days and twenty-five minutes* (264.4 hours), breaking the previous record of 260 hours (just over ten days) held by Tom Rounds. However, the Guinness Book of Records no longer recognizes periods of staying awake as world record attempts due to the unethical nature of people deferring sleep for long periods of time and the ill health they potentially would suffer as a result.

Whilst acute sleep loss tends to be linked to temporary life or work stressors, has minimal negative effects and can be overcome relatively easily, sleep debt is accumulative. Chronic sleep loss can have devastating effects, both physiologically and psychologically. It is no coincidence that sleep deprivation is used as a torture technique; without sleep, a person will feel awful. Any reader who, for example, is a new parent or perhaps works shifts or has had a new pet to house-train will identify with the feelings of chronic poor sleep and how dreadful it can make one feel on a day-to-day basis.

If sleep is restricted, an individual will suffer short- and long-term consequences, such as impaired thought processes, decreased reaction times, drowsiness, irritability, poor decision making and a general decrease in motivation to complete activities requiring focus. Most alarmingly, there is an increased susceptibility to numerous diseases, such as cardiovascular disease, Alzheimer's, diabetes and certain cancers (Cherpak & Van Lare, 2019). Sometimes clinical intervention is required for chronic sleep loss as there may be a sleep or circadian rhythm disorder present.

With regard to the negative consequences of poor sleep, consider for a moment the 2001 UK Selby rail crash where a Land Rover Defender, driven by a 37-year-old man and towing a loaded trailer (carrying a car), left the carriageway of the westbound M62 motorway and travelled 27 metres down an embankment, landing on the southbound railway track. Unfortunately, the Land Rover was hit by a southbound Great North Eastern Railway Intercity 225 heading from Newcastle to London. This train was then tragically deflected into the path of an oncoming Freightliner freight train (Health and Safety Executive, 2002). Sadly, ten people were killed, including the drivers of both trains, and 82 were seriously injured. The cause was found to be a result of driving in a sleep-deprived state on the part of the Land Rover driver, who had been up the previous night talking on the telephone to a woman he had met through an internet dating agency. It remains the worst rail disaster of the 21st century in the UK and a perfect example of the disregard for lack of sleep and levels of alertness when considering driving a car.

According to the Department of Transport, sleepiness whilst driving may be a contributory factor in as many as 20 per cent of all road accidents (Jackson et al., 2011). High-risk groups for road traffic accidents whilst tired include young (male) drivers, shift workers and professional

drivers or drivers of commercial vehicles. This highlights the importance of having industry standards relating to managing sleep. Table 2.3
displays the situations in which crashes caused by tired drivers are most
likely to happen (Royal Society for the Prevention of Accidents, 2024)
and emphasizes the importance of not driving if feeling at all sleepy.

Table 2.3 Situations in which crashes caused by tired drivers are most likely to happen (Royal Society for the Prevention of Accidents, 2024)

Most likely situations
On long journeys on monotonous roads, such as motorways
Between midnight and 6 a.m. or between 2 p.m. and 4 p.m. (especially after eating, or having even one alcoholic drink)
After having less sleep than normal after drinking alcohol
If taking medicines that cause drowsiness
After long working hours or on journeys home after long shifts, especially night shifts

Sleep therefore is a non-negotiable state, and the good news is that sleep
is free, readily available and can be described as the ultimate performance enhancer. I often refer to it as 'the not-so-secret secret weapon'.
That is, everyone knows about sleep, it's no secret – we all do it and
know how much better we feel after a good night's sleep. Yet those
individuals who adopt a sleep health strategy and consider their sleep,
prioritize it, value it and personalize their sleep window are the people
who will more likely perform better in daily life activities. They have the
secret weapon to 'wellness' if you will. They are the ones who are more
productive in the workplace and feel happier and healthier as a result
of good sleep. Indeed, the simple truth is that sleep is an individual
process, and the human species absolutely needs it, every day. It is a
universal process – everyone does it and without it human beings would
die. It is therefore arrogant to assume that people can defy evolution
and thrive on shorter, disturbed rest, which is an unfortunate reality in
many modern civilizations (Wallop, 2014).

HOW DO HUMANS FALL ASLEEP?
(SLEEP REGULATION)

Now we have looked at what human sleep is in terms of the 'timeout' it offers the human body and brain from being awake, let's consider how a person falls and stays asleep. Given the significance of sleep to sustain basic human life, it is important to understand how it is *regulated*. Most people wouldn't know what is happening in their body at the exact moment they fall asleep, and the reason for that lies deep within the brain.

Sleep is essentially a balance mechanism (Fullagar *et al.*, 2015). The process of physiological balance maintenance is termed 'homeostasis' and controls basic human function. That is, the human body operates in relatively stable equilibrium (homeostasis) for all manner of physiological processes, and if the internal physiological state becomes unbalanced, even ever so slightly, then the body responds accordingly. For example, the human body works to maintain its core body temperature (typically 36.5–37.5 °C), appetite and hormone release on a continuous basis. It doesn't operate well if it becomes too hot or cold, too hungry or full, or with a hormone imbalance. Sleep helps humans manage the equilibrium and maintains the body's status quo as it constantly adjusts for survival.

On a very basic level, sleep is a process involving several biological factors: the body's need to maintain homeostasis (physiological balance), neurophysiological control (nervous system) and an element of automaticity (sleep is a spontaneous action which is paid little attention to). How these elements all interact influences the regulation of sleep. Figure 2.2 illustrates the basic anatomy of the brain as a useful reference point for some aspects of this chapter's descriptions of sleep regulation.

Borbély's (1982) two-part model of sleep involving two processes – Process-S and Process-C – is widely regarded as the most influential theory of the regulation of sleep (Gandhi *et al.*, 2015). Put simply, it describes the regulatory homeostatic drive for sleep (Process-S) and the body's circadian rhythm (Process-C), which are independent but work synergistically. The model hypothesizes how sleep regulation is achieved through Process-S (homeostasis) responding to internal cues for sleep need and Process-C (circadian rhythm) responding to external cues. The model involves an arousal system which promotes wakefulness and, when its processes are inhibited, encourages sleep.

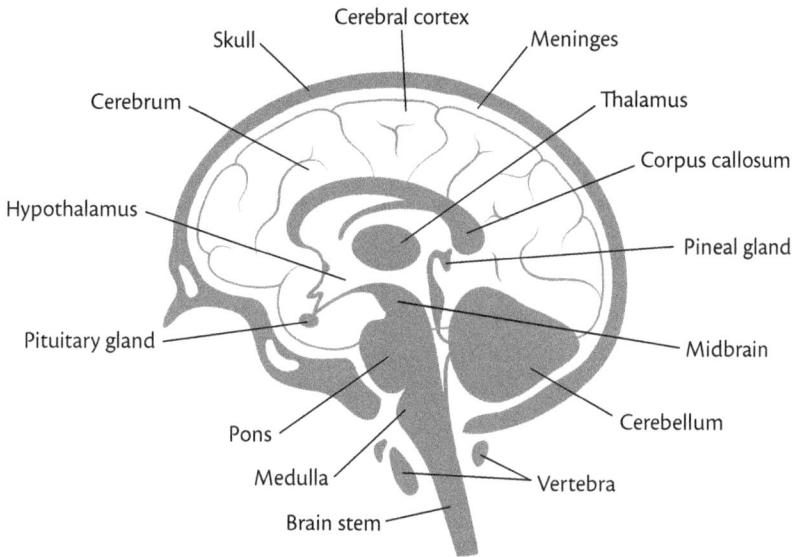

FIGURE 2.2 ANATOMY OF THE BRAIN

SLEEP PRESSURE

Process-S describes the sleep pressure (sometimes referred to as 'sleep drive') which builds throughout the waking day and involves the *ascending arousal system* (AAS) and its interaction with the sleep-inducing *ventrolateral preoptic nucleus* (VLPO); the former governs wakefulness, and the latter responds to sleep cues. This is a complex system of neurocircuitry and beyond the scope of this book, but I will describe the two-part process by means of an introductory technical description of sleep regulation.

The AAS has a subcortical (below the cerebral cortex[3]) neural circuitry, which is discrete yet mutually dependent on the circuitry for wakefulness, and is essential to consciousness. The AAS includes numerous neurons involved with various neurotransmitters,[4] such as serotoninergic (serotonin) and dopaminergic (dopamine), which are located in the upper brain stem. Projections from these numerous cell groups fire in a distinctive pattern to promote arousal. The AAS neurons project

---

3   The cerebral cortex is the outer layer of the brain. It is the centre of conscious thought, memory recall and behaviour. It is shown in Figure 2.2.
4   Neurotransmitters are chemical messengers that facilitate communication between neurons in the brain and nervous system.

and connect the brain stem to other key brain regions (such as the thalamus, hypothalamus, basal forebrain and cortex), activating awareness networks throughout the cerebral cortex. The AAS promotes wakefulness through these various projections, which characteristically 'fire' when homoeostatic and circadian drive (more of which shortly) dictate wakefulness (Schwartz & Roth, 2008). This is when sleep pressure is seen to be low, typically in the morning following a bout of nighttime sleep.

Conversely, the AAS is inhibited by sleep-promoting neurons every 24 hours from the ventrolateral preoptic nucleus (VLPO). This is a small cluster of neurons housed in the hypothalamus. Facilitators of the VLPO are several but, predominantly, it is activated by the *sleep-inducing* neurotransmitters serotonin and adenosine. The VLPO is inhibited during wakefulness by the *arousal-inducing* neurotransmitters noradrenaline and acetylcholine. It is the interaction between the VLPO and the AAS pathway which acts like an 'on–off' switch for sleep, thus enabling the body to maintain a homeostatic state. The VLPO is activated when sleep pressure is high, often in the evening when one is ready for sleep.

As the human body thrives in a well-balanced state, the longer it is in a state of wakefulness, the more the drive to maintain the body's homeostatic state is enhanced and the pressure to fall asleep increases. This urge to sleep increases linearly the longer one remains awake and then decreases during sleep (Schwartz & Roth, 2008). In terms of what is happening in the brain to cause sleep pressure to increase, it is a fight between the *sleep-promoting centre* (VLPO) and *arousal centre* (AAS) (wakefulness). In a healthy adult, sleep pressure is typically at its highest point in the late evening and lowest point early in the morning, and is dictated somewhat by the amount of preceding sleep an individual has achieved.

The abrupt nature of the transition between sleep and wakefulness is linked to the mutual inhibitory exchange between the AAS and sleep-inducing VLPO. This exchange acts as a feedback loop and is described, in electrical circuitry terminology, as a bistable 'flip-flop' circuit in which the two halves strongly inhibit one another – that is, they are either 'on' or 'off'. There is minimal time spent in a 'transitional' state and therefore, changes between the two states are quick (Schwartz & Roth, 2008). In short, sleep regulation involves the swift 'flip-flop' action of the transition between sleep and wakefulness, and it is the action of the VLPO which promotes sleep through its inhibition of the AAS.

CIRCADIAN RHYTHMS

Working synergistically with sleep pressure, but not related physiologically, is the internal *circadian rhythm* and its relationship to the light–dark cycle and sleep. Responding to external cues, such as cycles of light and dark over a 24-hour period, many aspects of human biology have a circadian rhythm – for example, core body temperature, appetite and immune function. Besedovsky *et al.* (2012) reported the sleep–wake cycle as being the most 'prominent manifestation of the circadian rhythm'. It is the misalignment of the sleep circadian rhythm which causes jet lag, a temporary condition caused by travelling quickly over several time zones.

The process aiding the circadian rhythm associated with light and dark (or sleep and wake) is governed through a biological component, the *suprachiasmatic nucleus* (SCN). This is a very important part of human biology as, located deep in the brain in the hypothalamus, it is the 'central governor' of all human circadian rhythms. If you hold a pencil between your eyes and ears and point it into your head, this would be roughly where you'd find this tiny but incredibly important aspect of human biology. This biological boss of all cells ensures synchronicity of any cell, using a rhythm to help its function. Now, that's a lot of cells!

With reference to sleep, the circadian rhythm uses external cues through the retina, which houses specialized light-sensitive (*photosensitive*) cells that send signals via the retinohypothalamic tract (RHT)[5] to the SCN. The photosensitive light receptors in the eye filter light through to the SCN and work in conjunction with the body's ascending arousal system (Process-S) to ensure sleep and wakefulness occur in response to the light and dark cues (Process-C). So external cues work in conjunction with the body's sleep and wake systems to ensure a person sleeps or wakes in response to the external light and dark signals (Process-C). The whole process is one long cascade system. Involved in this interconnecting system of neural circuitry and homeostatic and circadian rhythm is an endocrine[6] element (hormone signalling), which uses

---

5   The retinohypothalamic tract is a photic (light) neural input pathway involved in the circadian rhythms of mammals. It originates in the retinas of the eyes and travels to the hypothalamus deep in the brain.

6   The endocrine system is a network of glands and organs located throughout the body. It uses chemical messengers called hormones to regulate a range of bodily functions through the release of such hormones.

certain hormones to communicate and signal wakefulness in response to light and sleep in response to dark (Borbély, 1982).

Produced in the pineal gland in the brain, a principal hormone in this sleep-signalling process is the hormone *melatonin*. I often refer to this as the 'Dracula hormone', because plasma melatonin levels peak at night (Cherpak & Van Lare, 2019). It is a naturally occurring hormone and is strongly associated with the regulation, signalling and quality of human sleep. It is released in the evening in response to low light levels (<30–50 lux) and via stimulation from the SCN. Typically, melatonin levels take approximately two hours to reach peak levels and it interacts with sleep regulatory systems to ensure sleep ensues. It essentially inhibits the circadian drive for wakefulness after receiving information that light is fading (Process-C). Bright light is effectively the 'sleep robber', given its effect on melatonin release.

Daylight helps alertness as it sends signals to the SCN that light is abundant and thus melatonin is suppressed. A person will remain alert and awake until nighttime ensues and dim light means melatonin is stimulated once more. Exposure to too much bright light in the evening suppresses the release of melatonin, which has a resultant effect on an individual's ability to fall asleep at an appropriate time in the evening. Melatonin secretion is one of the principal reasons why a regular sleep schedule is important.

In summary, Borbély's (1982) two-part model of sleep regulation describes the activities over a 24-hour period, where, throughout the day, there is a rise in homeostatic sleep drive, coupled with a decline in the circadian signal for wakefulness, accompanied by the release of melatonin as light fades.

It should be noted that in the UK, melatonin is classified as a medication and is only available to purchase after receiving a prescription from a doctor or a registered prescriber. It is commonly used in other countries (as a prescription or over-the-counter medicine) as a means to combat jet lag symptoms, although its effectiveness is debatable and other, more practical strategies may be equally of use. There are also contraindications to using melatonin which should be considered before its use, so advise your clients to get some guidance from a GP. More information on sleep supplements is provided in Chapter 9.

Before we move on from the circadian rhythm and sleep, it's pertinent to mention daylight saving time or the 'spring forward' and 'fall back' clock change. This occurs twice a year, in the UK at one in the morning on the third Saturday in March (spring forward) and two in the morning, six months later, on the final Saturday in October (fall back). The clock change can be a major disrupter of sleep for some people, mainly due to the misalignment of their natural sleep rhythm, either forwards or backwards depending on the time of year. This misalignment can have a knock-on effect on an individual's productivity in the subsequent days as they readjust following the loss or gain of an hour's sleep over the weekend. In particular, the darker mornings and loss of an hour's sleep in the spring means it is harder to adjust to the spring-forward clock change. Moving the clocks forward creates a 'phase delay' in the body's innate natural circadian rhythm and it becomes at odds with the extrinsic environmental clock.

JET LAG

A brief note on jet lag as it is so intrinsically linked to the circadian rhythm's synchronicity with light and dark. Jet lag is a desynchronization of an individual's circadian rhythms caused by crossing multiple time zones in a relatively short time frame. Like sleep, jet lag is individualized, with some individuals experiencing worse jet lag symptoms than others, depending on the number of time zones crossed. Typical symptoms are daytime sleepiness, difficulty sleeping at night, problems with concentration and focus, and a disrupted mood.

The best way to overcome jet lag is to realign the body clock to the new time zone as soon as possible. The quickest and most straightforward way to do this is through using correct timing of exposure to sunlight and darkness and mealtimes in the new time zone. Most airlines these days have advice on their websites for the best way to combat jet lag depending on the direction one is travelling in and the length of the journey.

Historically, daylight saving time was introduced during the First World War in an effort to save energy (coal) by having lighter evenings. By moving the clocks forward in spring and back in autumn, people were able to make better use of daylight and reduce the need for artificial lighting in the evenings. This saved energy and, with fortuitous foresight, reduced environmental impact. Subsequently, this has become seasonal practice aimed at maximizing daylight hours and saving energy.

However, daylight saving is not practical or beneficial in modern industrialized societies, and there is an argument in contemporary societies for a permanent standard time to become the norm, which would be best aligned to human circadian rhythm and would have benefits for public health and safety.

Interestingly, only 70 out of 195 UN countries shift their time from international standard time. However, until such seasonal time-shift changes are universally obsolete, societies will have to manage around the twice-yearly change. The good news is that in the spring there are slightly darker mornings for a while so an individual may not be woken up quite as early, and the evenings are lighter, giving more opportunity for productivity, either professionally or from a personal point of view.

Nonetheless, recognize the effect of bright light on sleep (the sleep robber) and encourage your clients to make appropriate changes to help sleep – for example, eye masks in light evenings, and blackout blinds or curtains. It may be helpful in the preceding days before the spring-forward clock change to move bedtime earlier by approximately ten minutes a night, close curtains earlier, refrain from caffeine intake an hour earlier than normal, and reduce alcohol intake before bed. Similarly, when the clocks fall back in the autumn, it could be useful to adjust a sleep schedule to later than normal by about ten to fifteen minutes a night in the days preceding the clock change. A regular sleep routine should be emphasized in readjusting to a clock change, in addition to getting lots of natural daylight. Some of the practical tips outlined in Chapter 9 may also be beneficial in ensuring good sleep strategies.

GAMMA-AMINOBUTYRIC ACID (GABA)

Back to sleep regulation. Gamma-aminobutyric acid (GABA) is another central component to mention in the regulation of sleep. It is the main inhibitory neurotransmitter of the central nervous system (CNS), thus an influencer on sleep and relaxation, and it is well established that activation of GABA receptors favours sleep (Gottesmann, 2002; Cherpak & Van Lare, 2019). GABA neurones are also related to sleep spindle generation which, when sleep is monitored in a sleep laboratory, is an indicator of non-rapid eye movement (NREM) sleep, in particular stage 2 NREM sleep. Sleep architecture is the basic pattern of normal sleep and involves two main types, non-rapid eye movement and rapid eye movement sleep, and will be outlined in more detail later in this chapter.

GABA AND STRESS

GABA is linked to the stress hormone cortisol, since low levels of GABA mean an activated hypothalamic–pituitary–adrenal axis (HPA axis), which is a central player in the release of cortisol. The HPA axis is a three-component system made up of the hypothalamus, pituitary and adrenal glands, which, among other functions, play a crucial role in regulating stress responses in the body. Sleep restriction is a key stimulus for a stress response and activation of the HPA axis. This stimulus sets off a cascade of responses from the HPA with the hypothalamus releasing corticotropin-releasing hormone (CRH), which stimulates the pituitary gland to release adrenocorticotropic hormone (ACTH) into the bloodstream, which informs the adrenal glands to release the stress hormone cortisol (and other hormones). Elevated cortisol levels are also associated with sleep disturbance as an increase in cortisol will impair serotonin production, which is a precursor to production of melatonin, the hormone responsible for signalling sleep or waking states (Cherpak & Van Lare, 2019). This is a whole-body inflammatory response and operates as a positive feedback loop: unless the stress response subsides, cortisol levels remain elevated and build on the adverse consequences – for example, negative health states such as depression and anxiety. Figure 2.3 illustrates the hypothalamic–pituitary–adrenal axis (HPA) and its positive feedback loop.

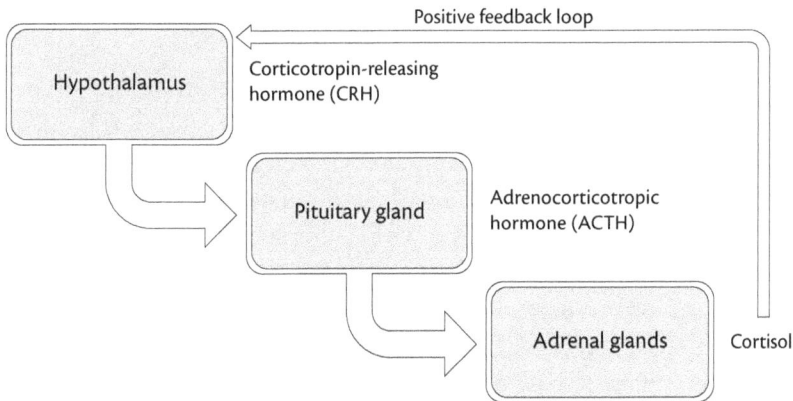

FIGURE 2.3 THE HYPOTHALAMIC–PITUITARY–ADRENAL AXIS (HPA) AND ITS POSITIVE FEEDBACK LOOP

Specifically relating to sleep, sustained stress increases cortisol levels and may induce sleep disorders, leading to impaired sleep quality and shortened sleep duration, with potential consequences to reproductive function as well as wider health issues (Cherpak & Van Lare, 2019; Beroukhim, Esencan & Seifer, 2022). There is more information on the HPA axis in later chapters as it can influence many aspects of a woman's sleep throughout her life. Suffice to say, reducing stress will have a positive impact on a woman's sleep quality and quantity.

One in four people in the UK state stress as a key factor in losing sleep. The factors that cause stress vary from person to person and the level of stress a person feels comfortable with may be higher or lower than that of others (National Health Service (NHS), 2024). Possible causes of stress can include (among others): genetics, upbringing and experiences as children or adults, personal problems such as relationship issues or pressure at school or home, or financial worries, housing issues and work problems (which is not surprising given the cost-of-living crisis at the time of writing) (NHS, 2024). Some of the practical strategies in Chapter 9 and resources at the end of this book may help if you have clients who are feeling stressed, which is then affecting their sleep (or vice versa, where poor sleep health is perhaps causing stress).

AUTOMATICITY

It is from an understanding of such physiological processes as homeostasis, circadian drive and neurophysiological circuitry that we can state that sleep is dominated by a physiological impetus. Yet it has a strong psychological component too. Known as automaticity, this psychological element of sleep helps make the case that sleep is a psycho-physiological process. 'Automatic' here means it occurs without conscious thought or attention. Good sleepers don't know how or why they fall asleep, they just do. Sleep for them is an automatic process, occurring involuntarily in a well-adjusted sleep schedule. Sleep requires no effort and occurs passively with persistent regularity. Where problems with automaticity of sleep arise, we see issues such as the sleep disorder insomnia. This ties in with my earlier point that no single scientific or medical domain owns sleep; it is highly complex and multidisciplinary in its manifestation.

Automaticity reinforces the view that those who are good sleepers do not necessarily know how they do it or why they find it easy, but essentially good sleep is not an issue for them. Sleep for these individuals is a normal routine, an automatic process, occurring involuntarily in a well-adjusted sleep routine. Sleep, for these fortunate people, requires no effort and occurs passively with determined regularity (Broomfield *et al.*, 2006). When this natural automated mode gets interrupted is when sleep disorders, such as insomnia, manifest (Broomfield *et al.*, 2006). Here sleep becomes the 'attention focus', and whilst sleep is important to those experiencing insomnia, it becomes less achievable as the person places excessive focus on, and experiences heightened anxiety about, sleep (Broomfield *et al.*, 2006). Other sleep disorders will affect automaticity too, and if this is the case, then you should advise that clients seek specialist, clinical sleep support.

In summary, sleep regulation is highly complex. It involves the body's need to maintain a fixed equilibrium, its responses to biological rhythms and a distinct and overriding electrophysiological structure. With its unique circuitry deep in the brain, the neurophysiology of sleep is the driving force behind the regulation of sleep and wakefulness. Extensive detail about the regulation of sleep is beyond the scope of this book, but it is hoped you now have a basic understanding of the processes governing how humans get to sleep; that there is a sleep pressure that builds throughout the day and helps an individual nod off when the need becomes too great. In line with this, there is a biological rhythm that interacts with light and dark cues and hormone secretion to help signal the body to be either awake or asleep. In essence, the basic human tendency to sleep is governed by the time passed since the previous sleep episode (homeostatic drive) and time of day (circadian drive) (Thun *et al.*, 2015). There is also an automatic process that means, in the absence of a sleep or circadian rhythm disorder, an individual will head off to sleep in a fairly automatic manner at the end of each day. For a more detailed look into the neurotransmitters involved in sleep regulation, I would urge you to look, in the first instance, at the *Oxford Handbook of Sleep Medicine* (Leschziner, 2022) and the extensive academic literature on the topic.

THE ARCHITECTURE OF SLEEP

Knowing about sleep-promoting and arousal systems, sleep pressure and the circadian rhythm of sleep and wakefulness helps us understand what happens pre-sleep and how it is regulated. But what happens when a person's eyes are shut and their head hits the pillow? What's going on when the lights are out? What happens *during* sleep is known as the *structure* or, more technically, the *architecture* of sleep.

It is easy to believe that sleep is essentially a calm, unconscious and passive process, something individuals do in a relaxed state. For whole-body voluntary actions, this is true. Humans lie down and fall asleep with minimal movement until wakening. Yet for the brain, sleep is anything but restful. This isn't to say the brain is in a state of chaos whilst a person sleeps, but it is by no means resting. Perhaps one of the reasons why, as a species, humans need to sleep with such regularity is in order to allow their brains the energy and time to conduct the various neurophysiological processes they undergo during sleep. In short, during sleep, the brain goes on a roller-coaster ride adventure.

How do we know what lies in store for the human brain during sleep? The answer lies in the measurement methodologies of sleep. The scientific way of measuring or analysing human sleep structure is in a sleep laboratory, hooked up to many electrodes covering an individual's face and head. This is known as polysomnography (PSG) and it is the gold-standard measurement technique of sleep quantity and quality. It is used primarily for assessing clinical sleep disorders, although it can be expensive and limited in its ability to measure large numbers of people due to being labour intensive and requiring specific skills in electrode placement and analysis of outputs.

Specifically, PSG can record body functions such as brain activity (electroencephalogram, EEG), eye movements (electrooculogram, EOG), muscle activity (electromyogram, EMG), and cardiac activity (electrocardiogram, ECG) (Halson, 2014). At a basic level, it can provide accurate information on useful sleep parameters such as total sleep time (TST), sleep efficiency (SE) (time asleep/time in bed), sleep onset latency, wake after sleep onset (WASO), sleep fragmentation index (FI), number of awakenings, time in each sleep stage and sleep stage percentages (Halson, 2014).

From laboratory studies using gold-standard PSG, we know that a human's sleep architecture typically comprises a 90-minute sleep cycle, consisting of four stages of sleep each with its own description and recognizable electrical brain wave patterns (EEG).

It was previously thought that humans had five stages of sleep during their 90-minute sleep cycle (Rechtschaffen & Kales, 1968); however, in 2004 the American Academy of Sleep Medicine replaced this with a four-stage classification system (Moser *et al.*, 2008; Gupta *et al.*, 2016).

As shown in Table 2.4, the first three stages of sleep involve non-rapid eye movement stages (NREM1, NREM2 and NREM3) and comprise the largest part of the sleep cycle, involving approximately 75 per cent of a healthy adult's nocturnal sleep bout. The term 'non-rapid eye movement' stems from research in sleep laboratories, where electrodes affixed onto a person's eyelids fail to record much eye movement in the first three stages of sleep, along with higher-amplitude, slow-frequency brain waves, particularly in stage 3 sleep. What makes stage 4 sleep distinct from the other three stages are characteristic fast, high-frequency brain waves, alongside rapid, horizontal eye movements, hence the term 'rapid eye movement' (REM) sleep.

The first few stages of sleep are a relatively short stepwise progression into deep sleep. Heart rate and breathing rate slow down, blood pressure decreases and a person will fall from a stage of light sleep (NREM1 and 2) into a deep sleep in stage 3 (NREM3).

It is in stages 1 and 2 sleep that napping is thought best to occur. These lighter stages of sleep in the first 15 to 30 minutes of the 90-minute sleep cycle mean the sleep inertia (grogginess) to overcome upon waking is far less than in deep, stage 3 sleep. So if you are going to suggest a nap to clients, make sure you advise one for either 20–30 minutes or 90 minutes to allow the individual to wake up in a lighter stage of sleep. More on napping, or, more specifically, sleep extension strategies, in Chapter 9.

Stage 3 sleep is also referred to as 'slow-wave sleep' (SWS) due to the slow brain waves seen during this stage of sleep, along with intense activity in certain parts of the brain. During this time, heart rate slows and blood pressure and breathing rate decrease. Longer periods of stage 3 sleep occur in the first part of the night, primarily in the first two sleep cycles, and it is recognized that this is an important stage of sleep for restoration and repair of muscle tissue, memory consolidation and cognitive recovery (Silva *et al.*, 2012). It is a fundamental part of the sleep cycle.

Table 2.4 The four stages of sleep

Stage	Description
Stage 1 (NREM1)	Transition to sleep
	Non-rapid eye movement sleep (NREM)
	Slow rolling eye movements
	Partial relaxation of voluntary muscles
	Relatively brief sleep stage (lasting up to seven minutes)
Stage 2 (NREM2)	Non-rapid eye movement sleep (NREM)
	The stage an individual ideally wakes in after a 'nap'
	Sleep spindles prevalent
Stage 3 (NREM3)	Non-rapid eye movement sleep (NREM)
	The start of deep sleep
	Shows high-amplitude activity (tall and wide brain waves) known as delta waves
	Reported as the deepest of the three NREM stages of sleep
	No eye movement or muscle activity
	Difficult to wake up in this stage of sleep (large sleep inertia)
Stage 4 (REM)	Rapid eye movement sleep (REM)
	Presence of rapid eye movement (REM) (the movement of eyes in different directions whilst you are asleep)
	Often referred to as the 'dream sleep stage'
	The average adult has 5–6 REM cycles per night.
	A deep stage of sleep with intense activity in certain parts of the brain. This is the phase when most dreaming occurs, heart rate and blood pressure increase, and breathing becomes fast, irregular and shallow.

The final stage of sleep (REM) is when most dreaming occurs, heart rate and blood pressure increase, and breathing becomes fast, irregular and shallow. It constitutes approximately 25 per cent of a healthy adult's nocturnal sleep bout and is more frequent during the latter stages of the night. It is thought this stage of sleep helps to ensure a person's emotional state is kept in balance (Takahashi et al., 1968). Without stage 4 sleep, people are less able to cope with the emotional demands placed on them during waking hours, their positive emotional state is compromised and life in general feels harder to manage. If a client comments on getting those days where things just seem harder to manage or cope with, then these are probably days preceded by a period of poor sleep and the old adage of 'getting an early night to feel better in the morning' really does help! It is this stage of sleep that is particularly negatively affected by drinking alcohol, even in small amounts. More on this in Chapter 9 when I explore nutrition and sleep.

> As stage 4 REM sleep is when most dreams occur, it is perhaps no coincidence that during this phase of sleep muscles are paralysed (apart from muscles for vital functions, such as cardiac, pulmonary and digestion), which is perhaps a protective mechanism against acting out dreams. However, there are rare incidents where this has not been the case and with extreme consequences. If you're particularly interested in this aspect of sleep and dreaming, then read Dr Guy Leschziner's fascinating book *The Man Who Tasted Words: Inside the Strange and Startling World of Our Senses* (Leschziner, 2022).

SLEEP SPINDLES

Sleep spindles are a particular pattern of brain wave that occur during healthy non-rapid eye movement sleep. Known for their unique shape (they look like bursts of activity), they are the hallmarks of NREM sleep, present in all NREM sleep stages, but most prominent in stage 2 sleep. Whilst it is not directly known what their function is, they are considered to be related to the consistency of sleep by reducing a person's responsiveness to external stimuli whilst asleep (sensory shutdown). In other words, they help a person stay asleep. They are also thought to be related to brain plasticity, the ability of the brain to reorganize its structure and function, and also linked to memory formation, learning and motor ability (Schönauer & Pöhlchen, 2018). They are measured by EEG through the gold-standard sleep measurement of polysomnography.

BRAIN WAVES

There are five types of brain waves measured through PSG, each relating to a different stage of sleep or wake. Each brain wave operates at a different frequency – for example, gamma waves are typically observed when a person is awake and operate at 31–100 Hz, whilst delta waves are associated with stage 3 sleep at a frequency of only 0.1–3 Hz. Figure 2.4

illustrates the different forms of brain waves observed and the level of awareness associated with each type.

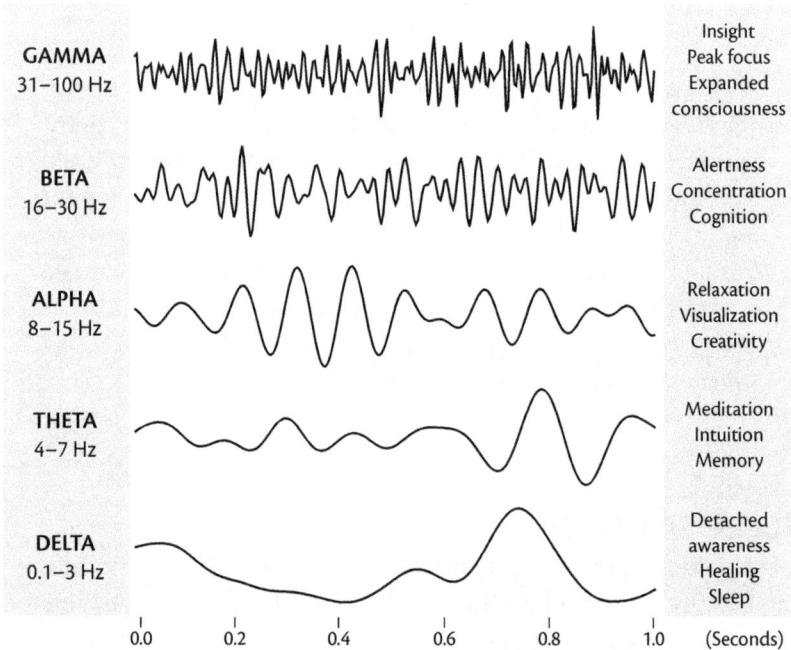

GAMMA 31–100 Hz		Insight Peak focus Expanded consciousness
BETA 16–30 Hz		Alertness Concentration Cognition
ALPHA 8–15 Hz		Relaxation Visualization Creativity
THETA 4–7 Hz		Meditation Intuition Memory
DELTA 0.1–3 Hz		Detached awareness Healing Sleep

0.0   0.2   0.4   0.6   0.8   1.0   (Seconds)

FIGURE 2.4 HUMAN BRAIN WAVES

HYPNOGRAMS

In analysing sleep architecture, if you were to summarize a night's assessment of sleep from polysomnography data, there would be hundreds of brain waves to decipher. Therefore, sleep scientists summarize the brain waves into a plot called a *hypnogram*. Measuring brain waves every 30 seconds, hypnograms are not the most accurate form of sleep analysis but they do allow a basic visualization of the structure of a person's sleep bout. Hypnograms are a useful way of observing the typical pattern of healthy sleep with more NREM sleep stages in the earlier part of the night and more REM sleep stages in the latter.

A hypnogram highlights the importance of the recommendation of having a regular sleep schedule, so as to ensure an individual is allowing themselves adequate sleep time to achieve enough sleep cycles (approximately four or five a night with sufficient time for NREM and REM components). For example, regularly getting up excessively early will short-change a person's ability to gain adequate REM sleep. Chapter 3 will look into sleep quantity and explore in more detail how much sleep a healthy adult needs over the course of a lifespan.

Hopefully, by now you have a sound understanding of the regulation of sleep, its two-part process involving homeostasis and circadian rhythms, and the architecture of sleep, with its cycling through the four sleep stages during a bout of nocturnal sleep. Key players supporting the regulation and architecture of sleep are GABA, sleep spindles and the body's stress responses.

OTHER OBJECTIVE METHODS OF SLEEP MEASUREMENT

Whilst objective assessment of sleep requires specific training and sometimes referral to a clinical sleep unit for PSG measurement of sleep, it's important for the reader's general understanding, and also for when I introduce in Chapter 9 some of the sleep aids available, to know of the different sleep assessment methods.

Clinically two common methods exist to measure sleep quality and quantity, the aforementioned gold-standard methodology of PSG and, second, actigraphy. Actigraphy is a non-invasive method of monitoring human rest/activity cycles. Devices house an accelerometer which is worn on the wrist or ankle and measures movement. Whilst PSG provides the most valid and reliable marker of sleep architecture, actigraphy is a more ecologically valid field measure of sleep quantity, quality and activity (Sadeh & Acebo, 2002; Ekblom *et al.*, 2012; Lambiase *et al.*, 2014). This is the technology I used in my doctorate and my work supporting elite athletes to optimize their sleep.

At the time of my sleep projects in elite sport, these actigraphy units were routinely used by sleep scientists. It is a popular choice for assessing sleep (and activity levels) in the field as it is validated against the benchmark PSG measurement and is a simple, relatively non-invasive method of monitoring human rest and activity cycles. A big advantage over PSG sleep assessment is that it allows sleep to be assessed in an individual's natural environment. Sadeh (2011) reported in a review of the role and validity of actigraphy that it has reasonable validity and reliability in normal individuals with relatively good sleep patterns. Compared to PSG, the gold-standard measurement of sleep, actigraphy has an accuracy of up to 80 per cent for the sleep markers of total sleep time and sleep efficiency in sleep disorder patients (Kushida *et al.*, 2001).

Whilst the two methods cannot directly be compared due to methodological differences, actigraphy at least is the preferred field measure over PSG due to its relative ease of use and cost-effective benefits, not just financially, but also for the subject's time (in my case, the athlete).

Other advantages of actigraphy is the discreet and compact design of the device, making wearing it easy and unobtrusive. Its placement involves a small actigraph unit (43 mm x 23 mm x 10 mm and 16 grams), which houses small uniaxial accelerometers (preferably 3 axes to be medically valid against PSG), and is usually intended to be worn on the wrist of the non-dominant arm to measure gross motor activity. The placement on the wrist makes it possible to study low-intensity physical activities as well as monitoring physical activity during sleep for sleep duration and quality assessment (Ekblom *et al.*, 2012).

However, there are some disadvantages to actigraphy technology in that its validity has not been established for all scoring algorithms or devices (typically 2-axis devices), nor for all clinical groups (Sadeh & Acebo, 2002). Also, it is not sufficient for diagnosis of sleep disorders in individuals with motor disorders or high motility during sleep.

Further, the two sleep assessment technologies may recognize sleep onset at different points. Tryon (1996) presented a spectrum for the onset of sleep to emphasize the organized nature of sleep onset and illustrate that sleep onset is a gradual rather than a isolated process. In the report, actigraphy was theoretically associated with Sleep Onset Spectrum phase 1 'quiescence' and PSG theoretically associated with Sleep Onset Spectrum phase 2, 'dropping handheld objects'. This makes direct comparisons in sleep onset through using the two methods difficult. Further, this difference is more pronounced in those with insomnia than normal sleepers (Tryon, 1996).

Finally, actigraphy relies on algorithms and, as with any computer-generated outcome, the use of computer scoring algorithms without controlling for potential sleep interferences can lead to inaccurate and misleading results. Nonetheless, the American Academy of Sleep Medicine accept validated actigraphs as an acceptable measure of total sleep time in certain circumstances (Byrne, 2017).

Another method for recording sleep is through subjective methodologies. This type of sleep assessment can be problematic in terms of overestimating sleep duration and accuracy of reporting, but it is also the most efficient, inexpensive, simple to administer and useful method for large-scale population assessment of sleep quality and quantity. Further, many self-assessment sleep questionnaires have high internal consistency (measure what they need to measure) and test–retest reliability (consistency over time) (Fabbri *et al.*, 2021).

The Pittsburgh Sleep Quality Index (PSQI) (Buysse *et al.*, 1989) is a popular self-assessment sleep questionnaire but others are available – for example, the Athens Insomnia Scale (AIS), Insomnia Severity Index (ISI), Mini-Sleep Questionnaire (MSQ), Jenkins Sleep Scale (JSS), Leeds Sleep Evaluation Questionnaire (LSEQ), SLEEP-50 Questionnaire, and Epworth Sleepiness Scale (ESS) (Fabbri *et al.*, 2021). The latter can be used independently from a technical sleep expert as this is simple scoring system providing an indication of daytime sleepiness. However, unless specifically trained, it would not be for you as a practitioner to administer most of these self-assessment sleep questionnaires to your clients. Nonetheless, it is important to have an understanding of the range available.

Other subjective methods to monitor a person's sleep include sleep diaries, which are reliable, cost-efficient and easy to administer to individuals or large groups of people to assess sleep quality and quantity. They consist of daily recording of information by an individual about their sleep habits, wakefulness and general activities over a certain number of days (de Alcantara Borba *et al.*, 2020). They can be a useful tool for reporting sleep quality and quantity and a valuable intelligence-gathering method for sleep issues. This is particularly useful if there is a requirement to see a healthcare professional, as the evidence of sleep–wake patterns that the diaries help produce can help with diagnosis and treatment. The sleep diaries are beneficial in identifying if an individual is consistently waking at a similar time, what daily activities they have taken part in, what they've eaten and so on, and help ascertain if there is any pattern to sleep disturbances. If using a sleep diary, then ideally advise clients to start keeping the diary as soon as they begin to recognize a problem with their sleep and complete it over a period of at least seven days. The Sleep Charity have an online sleep diary which is freely available and signposted at the end of this book.

After a heavy technical chapter, the next chapter will focus on sleep and ageing. As a practitioner, you may have observed age-related differences in your clients as they are likely to span several age groups. This next chapter will describe the start of differences in sleep between genders and the journey of sleep over the course of a woman's lifespan.

CHAPTER 3

Sleep and Age

I expect your clients report days when they wake up and feel like they've had a really restful night's sleep, 'a good deep sleep', and can tackle anything throughout the day. Then sometimes they wake up and feel awful; sleep wasn't overly restful for them and they could really do with staying in bed for longer! Sound familiar? How much sleep a person needs changes as they age, and sleep quantity is becoming more and more recognized as a specific need, and therefore the individual nature of sleep is becoming more evident in society (Chennaoui *et al.*, 2015).

Sleep evolves over a human's lifetime and not always to a person's advantage, as we will see throughout this book. From a woman's perspective, sleep certainly does change with age, and I will elaborate how as we travel through a woman's lifespan over the course of this book.

In relation to sleep and age, the questions I get asked most often are: why do we sleep less as we age and why do my teenagers not want to get up in the morning! The answer is simple: 'It's our biology!' Here's why.

From foetus to childhood, sleep undergoes many developmental changes which then continue into adult life. Significant changes in the time spent asleep, the pattern of sleep across a 24-hour period, the division of sleep stages, and an individual's sleep structure are observed from newborns through to adulthood (MacLean, Fitzgerald & Waters, 2015). What doesn't change, however, is the individuality of sleep. In Chapter 2, Table 2.1 highlighted the changes in sleep requirement over a person's lifetime, with indications of 'recommended' and 'maybe appropriate' sleep durations. Sleep windows outside of these parameters are not recommended. What Table 2.1 highlights is that whilst there are sleep recommendations, what works for one person may be very different for another of the same age.

CHILDHOOD SLEEP

Typically, as neonates, humans are predisposed to needing lots of sleep, and those early newborn days, snuggled up between feeds and nappy changes, are precious moments for baby (and parents), as well as a biological need. On the whole, newborns up to (approximately) two months old require 12 to 18 hours' sleep a day and this then gradually declines as they develop into preschool and then school-age children, who need approximately nine to 11 hours' sleep. As children develop into adolescence, they typically need eight and a half to nine and a half hours of sleep.

It's important to note that up until adolescence there is little difference in gender sleep patterns. From the information in Chapter 2 on sleep structure, you will have gathered that sleep is a highly complex state, involving interaction between multiple brain regions, nerve pathways and hormones. This complexity makes sleep highly vulnerable to disruption, and as a result, small changes in the brain during development, such as in adolescence, can have a significant impact upon sleep (Kelley *et al.*, 2015).

In terms of adolescent sleep and the circadian rhythm, what is common to both genders is that during the teenage years, the circadian clock shifts to a slightly later rhythm, therefore delaying the timing of when sleep can be initiated and prolonging wakefulness into the later evening. This is known as having an 'eveningness' tendency and is why teenagers are more likely to be awake later in the day and sleep longer into the next morning.

The sleep drive I mentioned in Chapter 2 also alters throughout the adolescent phase in that the sleep pressure build-up is slower in the teenage years and the aforementioned 'flip-flop switch' between awake and sleep takes longer to achieve, meaning a later time to sleep. This can make 'choosing' to go to sleep difficult for teenagers as the brain is still in a state where it is promoting wakefulness rather than sleep (Kelley *et al.*, 2015).

This isn't to say that a teenager's habit of staying up late at night 'gaming' or on social media isn't a bad habit to fall into, but the flip side of the coin is that teenagers are biologically programmed to be alert later within the normal 24-hour period than their typically middle-aged parents. Whilst gender differences in sleep disturbance start to appear in adolescence, the slight shift in circadian rhythm is common to both genders. Many of your clients who are parents of teenagers will be familiar with the 'before-school argument', where early school times are the predominant logistical problem with a sleepy teenager. It is not just a case of 'lazy' teenager. Biology does at least provide some explanation as to why young people turn into night owls during their adolescent years (Kirshenbaum *et al.*, 2023; Winnebeck, 2024). The social side of the matter is the challenge of parenting a teenager and beyond the focus of this book!

Throughout childhood, sleep quantity remains relatively stable; suffice to say, children still need significantly more than the average healthy adult. Only once puberty begins do we see a separation of sleep disturbances related to gender, with female sleep being inextricably linked with the cyclical monthly ovarian hormone release. Certainly, women of reproductive age experience more sleep disturbance than men, leading to a lack of restorative sleep and increasing the risk of chronic disease (Cherpak & Van Lare, 2019). More on this in Chapters 4, 5 and 6.

SLEEP FOR ADULTS AND OLDER AGE

As we learnt in Chapter 2, most healthy adults require seven to nine hours of sleep per night (in the absence of a sleep or circadian rhythm disorder), which is the suggested amount to reduce morbidity and mortality risks. This equates to four to six sleep cycles per night. As adults enter old age, this declines slightly, although it is a common misconception that sleep *needs* decline with age. It's not about requiring less sleep, but that unfortunately, as a person ages, sleep *quality* declines and an individual will experience a change in their sleeping patterns. For example, they are likely to experience more frequent night wakenings and lose some NREM stage 3 sleep (deep sleep), which means sleep can be less refreshing and restorative.

Further, exposure to daylight can be affected in older age as an individual may be less likely to engage in outdoor activities, possibly due to being less mobile. Ageing also means a person is less sensitive to light changes than in earlier adulthood and therefore experience a less robust circadian rhythm and sleep drive (Li *et al.*, 2022). A reduction in light exposure and a diminished response to light affects the circadian rhythm and its relationship with the light–dark cycle, as described in Chapter 2.

Studies have also shown that changes in production of hormones, such as melatonin, may play a role in disrupted sleep in older adults.

As people age, the body secretes less melatonin, which, as we learnt in Chapter 2, is normally produced in response to darkness and helps promote sleep by coordinating circadian rhythms. As a consequence, in older age, people tend to have earlier bed and wake-up times. This is known as phase advanced sleep. Whilst the circadian rhythm relating to the sleep–wake cycle normalizes in adulthood, it alters again in later life where there is a greater orientation towards morningness, which is obviously at odds with the aforementioned adolescent 'eveningness'.

Older people also display differences in sleep spindle activity which, with age, tends to occur less often and have a smaller frequency and duration. You may recall from Chapter 2 that sleep spindles help an individual stay asleep. Sleep spindle form tends to change across the lifespan, with sleep spindle density increasing throughout early development, peaking during puberty and steadily declining from adolescence to old age. Duration of sleep spindles also peaks early in life, and then generally declines over the lifespan, whilst spindle amplitude is relatively small in early years development, increasing to maximum values over the first year of life, and then steadily declines until old age (Clawson, Durkin & Aton, 2016). Reduced spindle activity has implications for memory and learning, which may have a concomitant effect on certain disease states in later life, such as Alzheimer's disease.

Overall, typical sleep changes in ageing involve a decreased total nocturnal sleep time, delayed onset of sleep, an advanced circadian phase (early to bed, early to rise), reduced slow-wave sleep (NREM3), reduced rapid eye movement sleep (REM) and a reduced threshold for arousal from sleep. Therefore, older people find it harder to get good-quality deep sleep and wake up more easily. They may also experience more fragmented (restless) sleep with multiple arousals – for example, due to other age-related factors such as an increase in nighttime urination. Daytime napping is also more likely, which may impact on nighttime sleep. The good news is that most age-related changes in sleep are stable after 60 years of age among older adults with good levels of health. Where sleep problems arise in later life, it is typically due to multifactorial reasons and not necessarily explained by age alone (Li *et al.*, 2022).

The main point to remember with sleep and ageing, for both genders, is that there are subtle changes over time and sleep remains an individual process. For the purposes of this book, I will now just focus on women's sleep over time.

CHRONOTYPE

A person's chronotype is very much linked to their circadian rhythm and sleep–wake cycle. Chronotype refers to the adage of whether they're a lark (morning person), an owl (evening person) or somewhere in between, and may also play a part in ageing and sleep. Roughly a third of the population are larks, a third owls and a third somewhere in between. Ask clients to take a look at their parents' sleep, or complete a simple online self-assessment questionnaire, such as the Morning-ness–Eveningness Questionnaire (MEQ) (Horne and Ostberg, 1976), if they are particularly interested in their chronotype. The main purpose of this questionnaire is to measure whether a person's circadian rhythm produces peak alertness in the morning, in the evening or in between. This can be useful information when discussing with clients their sleep scheduling and regular bed and get-up times, and to help provide effective sleep strategies. For example, a shift worker who is at the extreme spectrum of morning type may struggle with night shifts as their body won't like being awake so late in the day on a regular basis. Conversely, a night owl who is training for a marathon and only has time to train in the mornings may struggle to get up for regular early morning training runs. Most people tend to manage daily life around their chronotype due to responsibilities, commitments, type of employment and logistics, but it is always useful to be aware of chronotype for those instances when a client is an extreme 'type' and struggling with their sleep patterns.

The changes throughout life in the sleep circadian rhythm and structure are part of a human's normal, healthy development. Recognizing that alterations in sleep occur throughout life, and how to manage them, is half the battle in ensuring good sleep health for the majority of individuals. Of course, if there are comorbidities[1] or a suspected sleep or circadian rhythm disorder, advise clients to seek medical guidance.

---

1   Comorbidities are any coexisting health condition alongside a primary diagnosis and may affect a person's treatment and ongoing care. They are often chronic conditions and can include physical or mental health.

CHAPTER 4

Female Sleep Specifics: Puberty and the Menstrual Cycle

There has been plenty of focus on aspects of women's health over recent years. From menstruation to menopause, there are resources and information available across various media platforms, science, medicine, health and wellbeing outlets, and movements and organizations such as the Active Pregnancy Foundation, My Menopause Centre and Menopause Mandate to name a few.

However, what is not always commented on with regard to women's health over their lifespan is the impact of sleep. This is slightly shocking given that women are potentially more likely to suffer certain sleep disorders than men, such as insomnia. The good news is that, generally, sleep and sleep disturbances are increasingly recognized as determinants of a women's health and wellbeing, particularly in relation to the hormone transitions: menstrual cycle, pregnancy and menopause (Kloss *et al.*, 2015).

It's not surprising that a women's sleep is compromised. I talked briefly at the beginning of this book about how a woman's sleep is affected throughout her lifespan, and Figure 4.1 summarizes some of those areas. Whilst hormone transitions seem to be the predominant areas where a woman's sleep may be restricted, other aspects may also contribute, such as caregiving roles, performing shift work or living in pain. I'll explore each of these areas over the course of the next few chapters, and this should give you a more holistic view of a woman's relationship with sleep over the course of her lifetime and enable you to provide more informed support to your clients.

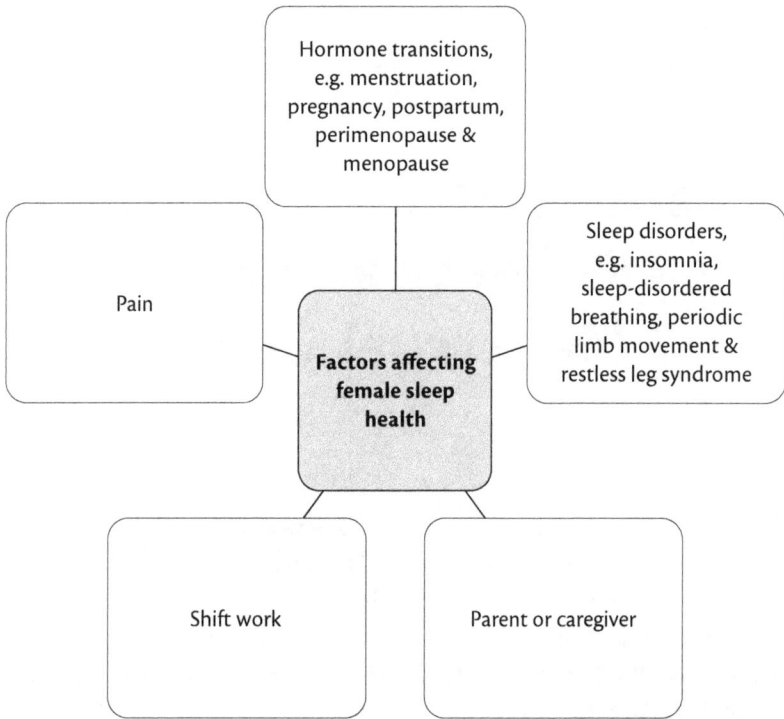

FIGURE 4.1 ASPECTS OF A WOMAN'S LIFE WHERE SLEEP MAY BE AN ISSUE

Delving into the world of women's sleep in the academic literature is not a simple exercise. There are multiple causes of sleep disturbances in women, but the pathophysiology is sometimes poorly understood (Haufe & Leeners, 2023). The complexity of the sleep process, combined with the parallel intricacy of the endocrine system, plus exogenous hormone options such as the oral contraceptive pill or hormone replacement therapy (increasingly prevalent in the menopause transition), means that assessment of sleep and female hormones is extremely challenging. Additionally, small sample sizes and methodological issues in research and the individual nature of sleep mean that making any conclusive findings around female sleep in relation to the hormone transitions of puberty, pregnancy and postpartum and the menopause transition is difficult and problematic.

Nevertheless, what is known is that sleep disturbances are common during the hormone transition stages of a woman's life and that levels of and changes in the reproductive hormones are likely to contribute to the sleep issues experienced (Haufe & Leeners, 2023).

That said, what I've tried to do over the next few chapters is provide an overview of the findings and explain the matter in a practical way that will help you open a dialogue with your clients around sleep in whatever phase of life they are in.

As a short summary of the changes in sleep over a woman's lifespan, Nowakowski *et al.* (2013), Pengo, Won and Bourjeily (2018) and Nowakowski (2021) provide some useful headlines. In childhood, no established gender differences in sleep exist, but in the reproductive years, factors during the menstrual cycle may disrupt sleep, and there is therefore more wake after sleep onset (WASO) time. More on this later in this chapter. In pregnancy, a woman may experience pregnancy-specific factors that disrupt sleep (more on this in Chapter 5), whereas in the menopause transition there is a myriad of sleep-affecting symptoms (more on this in Chapter 6). Finally, in ageing, a woman's sleep can potentially again be disrupted, with typically more WASO time and less total sleep time (TST) (Nowakowski *et al.*, 2013; Pengo *et al.*, 2018; Nowakowski, 2021).

This chapter will focus on the first stage of a woman's lifespan where gender differences around sleep are initially observed, and that is puberty. This is the earliest hormone transition in a woman's lifespan and a significant adjustment for a woman on many levels, including changes to her sleep health. Later chapters will focus on other hormone transitions, not forgetting the non-physiological aspects of a woman's lifespan where sleep may be affected.

A BRIEF NOTE ON HORMONES

Given the complexity of sleep and the relationship a woman's sleep has with her hormones over the course of a life cycle, let's focus on hormones for a short time. For health professionals reading this book, I'm going to assume some level of knowledge about endocrinology. However, as the term 'health professionals' tends to refer to a broad range of practitioners, I will provide a brief description of hormones and their relationship with sleep, as it is important to recognize this relationship when considering sleep health.

Sleep and hormones are intrinsically linked and it's not just sleep which can be complex. Hormones have traditionally been labelled as the body's 'chemical messengers', and whilst this is true, they are so much more than that. Dr Nicky Keay, a leading researcher in female hormone health, describes hormones beautifully as 'active participants in driving physiological processes that lead us to health' (Keay, 2022). They essentially bring deoxyribonucleic acid (DNA)[1] to life, as they inform DNA what to do in terms of an individual's response to something – for example, whether they need to cool down or warm up. Without hormones, a person wouldn't feel hungry, enjoy physical activity, or know when to wake up or fall asleep. Hormones essentially help a body react and prepare for anything it undergoes and maintain its coveted homeostatic or 'balanced' state. To do this, hormones require humans to have optimal behaviours around exercise, nutrition, recovery and sleep.

Like many aspects of human physiology, there is a bidirectional relationship between sleep and endocrine activity (Steiger, 2003). Various hormones influence sleep regulation, and a primary role is known for the reciprocal relationship between *sleep-promoting* growth hormone-releasing hormone (GHRH) (stimulates synthesis and release of growth hormone) and *sleep-impairing* corticotropin-releasing hormone (CRH)[2] which is involved in the body's stress responses. Alterations in the GHRH:CRH ratio result in changes of sleep-endocrine activity (Steiger, 2003), which can have implications for an individual's health, particularly as a chronic stress response (I briefly mentioned the body's stress response through the HPA axis in Chapter 2). Other hormones are linked to the regulation of sleep, and for women in particular, the ovarian hormones oestrogen and progesterone are thought to be associated with sleep regulation (Dorsey, De Lecea & Jennings, 2021).

Happy hormones help make the human body function well. Where there is an imbalance in behaviours, hormones are significantly challenged. For example, if a woman is exercising too much, eating too little and not sleeping enough, the internal body imbalance created from the

---

1   Deoxyribonucleic acid (DNA) – a compound contained in all the body's cells that directs cell activity.
2   Also known as corticotropin-releasing factor (CRF), whose main function is the stimulation of the pituitary gland to release corticotropic hormone (ACTH), as part of the hypothalamic–pituitary–adrenal axis (HPA axis).

energy deficit, high training load and lack of recovery will impact on the homeostatic balance of the physiological processes driving the hormones responsible for the menstrual cycle. In other words, her menstrual cycle will be disrupted. Those readers working in sport, supporting athletes, may have heard of the condition relative energy deficiency in sport (RED-S). This is a condition resulting from insufficient caloric intake and/or excessive energy expenditure which can affect athletes from recreational to elite. Suffice to say, this condition has a huge impact on the body's balanced state and hormone control of physiological function. More detail on this condition can be found in various outlets, but for a comprehensive guide refer to the International Olympic Committee (IOC) Consensus Statement on Relative Energy Deficiency in Sport (RED-S): 2018 Update (Mountjoy et al., 2018) and further articles in the British Journal of Sports Medicine – for example, Statuta et al., 2017.

Hormones are key to our bodies functioning, in the same way sleep is vital to human life. If you'd like more detail around hormones and women's health in general, then I'd urge you to look up papers by Professor Kirsty Sale and colleagues, which tend to focus on the menstrual cycle and exercise performance, alongside *Hormones, Health and Human Potential* (Keay, 2022), which is a fascinating read with some brilliant parallels of the human body's physiological processes to art and culture.

In these next few chapters, I provide an *overview* of the relationship between sleep and women's health at key points over the course of a lifespan. I am not suitably clinically qualified to go into detail regarding every female health complaint and its relationship with sleep. Some key conditions are good examples of how woman's sleep can be affected, such as pain from endometriosis,[3] but if you wish to explore female health conditions in more clinical detail, I urge you to look to the references provided, the wider academic literature and the relevant clinicians in the specialist areas. Signposting to organizations supporting women living with some of the conditions mentioned in the next few chapters is also provided at the end of this book.

---

3   Endometriosis is a condition where tissue similar to the lining of the womb grows in other places, such as the ovaries and fallopian tubes. It can affect women of any age and can be extremely painful (NHS, 2022).

PUBERTY AND SLEEP

Whilst sleep is a very dynamic process that changes every few weeks in one's early years, sleep differences between genders are negligible in the childhood years (Pengo *et al.*, 2018). As we learnt in the previous chapter, where sleep diverges between men and women is typically in the teenage years, once puberty sets in (Dorsey *et al.*, 2021).

Whilst sleep is good for the overall maintenance of hormone levels and, as a result, body homeostasis, sometimes hormones are responsible for upsetting this state of balance. For example, the reciprocal relationship between a woman's hormones and sleep is magnified once the first menstrual cycle has occurred. Without a doubt, once women begin menstruating and the ovarian hormones (oestrogen and progesterone) are released into their system, a dramatic difference in sleep between the genders is observed, and poor sleep during the menstrual cycle is a common complaint. What follows is a brief outline of the menstrual cycle to help inform an understanding of its relationship with sleep and how sleep health can be affected throughout it.

When considering the menstrual cycle, it is important to remember that, whilst it is a general biological process for all healthy reproductive women, each woman experiences it on an individual level. Female hormones have been described as having a remarkable and complicated synchronicity throughout the menstrual cycle, and each woman's hormone profile, and her responses to fluctuating hormones throughout the cycle, will be subtly different (Keay, 2022). Therefore, menstruation is a useful indicator of internal hormone health. If a woman is experiencing regular menstrual cycles, then one can assume body homeostasis is achieved. If there are irregularities associated with the menstrual cycle, then typically there could be internal or external issues impacting on its regular function. It is beyond the scope of this book to go into finite detail around the menstrual cycle, but a great resource for this is the aforementioned literature outputs by Professor Sale, McNulty PhD and Dr Keay.

THE MENSTRUAL CYCLE

Menarche is the phase of a woman's life when the menstrual cycle starts being active, ovarian function increases, the female hormones oestrogen and progesterone are cyclically released into the bloodstream and a healthy reproductive woman will experience a monthly 'bleed'.

The typical age in the UK to start menses (menstrual flow or a 'period') is 12 years old, although it could be slightly younger or older. If you know a client's periods have not begun by their 16th birthday, or you know they have an erratic menstrual cycle, then do advise that they speak to their GP. Also note that in female athletes, an erratic menstrual cycle could potentially be a sign of the previously mentioned relative energy deficiency in sport (RED-S), which requires clinical support.

The menstrual cycle consists of different components relating to a woman's health; key among these are cycle phase, hormone levels, uterine health and body temperature, all of which have a two-way relationship with sleep in some way. Menstrual cycle *phase* is fundamental and interacts with all the other components, so I will explain the relationship with sleep through the cycle phase model. This is from the perspective of a healthy menstruating woman and in the absence of any form of exogenous hormone supplementation.

Typically, a menstrual cycle in a healthy woman will last 28 days (but can range from 25 to 35 days) and is split into four distinct phases: (1) follicular (approximately days 1–14); (2) ovulation (approximately day 14), when the egg is released from the ovary; (3) luteal (approximately days 14–28); and (4) menses (approximately day 28). On average, a woman would have nine to 12 periods a year. Different ovarian hormones come into play at different stages of the cycle and there are four key hormones involved: follicle-stimulating hormone (FSH), luteinizing hormone (LH), oestrogen and progesterone, all of which have a rhythmic peak and trough throughout the cycle.

The cycle can be separated into two stages, the follicular, where oestrogen predominates, and luteal, where progesterone rules. Figure 4.2 shows the hormone profiles during the menstrual cycle. In the first half of the cycle, the ovaries are set to release an egg into a fallopian tube (ovulation). Oestrogen, FSH and LH levels rise in preparation for ovulation and decline once ovulation has occurred. It is at this point in the cycle that hormone interaction is determined, according to whether conception has occurred or not. If not, then progesterone levels rise in the luteal phase, with a concomitant second rise in oestrogen, which both then decrease as menses begins. The cycle then repeats itself once menses has finished for that month.

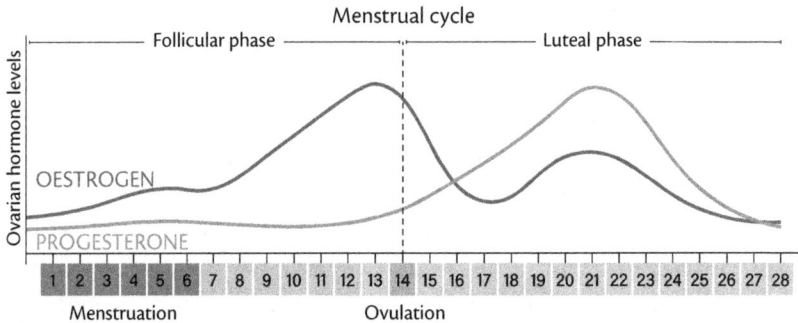

FIGURE 4.2 THE DIFFERENT PHASES OF THE MENSTRUAL CYCLE AND OVARIAN HORMONE LEVELS

There are many aspects of the menstrual cycle that interact with sleep, and the changes in sleep across the monthly cycle can be related to the four key ovarian hormones and the menstrual phase in which they occur. Generally, numerous sleep disturbances can be related to menses – for example, dysmenorrhea (painful menstrual periods) or heavy menstrual bleeding (Baek, 2023), ovulation, and in the post-ovulation (luteal) phase, when oestrogen and progesterone levels are high and many of the symptoms relating to premenstrual syndrome (PMS) predominate (more on premenstrual symptomology later in this chapter) (Dorsey *et al.*, 2021) – all of which can impact a woman's sleep (Xing *et al.*, 2020). This can even be the case for women without significant menstrual-related complaints (Nowakowski *et al.*, 2013).

Haufe and Leeners (2023), in their review of sleep disturbances across a woman's lifespan, stated that the earlier phases of the menstrual cycle (follicular and ovulatory) have been associated with longer periods of deep sleep compared with the stage around menstruation: perhaps a protective sleep mechanism ahead of the potential disturbed sleep during this time? Other studies have suggested influences on reproduction and menstrual cycle regularity, with raised FSH and LH levels in response to compromised sleep (Beroukhim *et al.*, 2022). Similarly, some studies have suggested an association between raised FSH levels and wakefulness, but these are sparse, and no specific measurements of FSH and LH and sleep have been published (Haufe & Leeners, 2023).

Throughout the literature, there is strong support for a regulatory role of the ovarian hormones oestrogen and progesterone in sleep–wake cycles across different species (Brown & Gervais, 2020). Both hormones are major players in the game of women's good sleep health (Pengo *et al.*, 2018; Brown & Gervais, 2022). As well as contributing to sleep–wake cycle regulation, they help to regulate a large variety of homeostatic functions, involving the cardio-circulatory, respiratory and metabolic systems (Pengo *et al.*, 2018). Oestrogen, for example, travels throughout the body via the bloodstream and affects bone health, mental health, soft tissue repair and digestion, in addition to its role in menstruation. However, there is no *specific* association between oestrogen and sleep during a woman's menstrual cycle.

On the other hand, progesterone has a strong link with sleep during the menstrual cycle where, in the luteal phase, a rise in progesterone causes an increased metabolic rate and elevated core body temperature, which has a concomitant effect on sleep (core body temperature needs to be on the decline to help an individual fall asleep) (Xing *et al.*, 2020). During the luteal phase there is a dramatic increase in stage 3 sleep brain wave activity (deep sleep), supposedly as a protection mechanism from the more restless sleep a woman may experience during this phase of her monthly cycle. As progesterone levels decline quite rapidly in the late luteal phase, some women report poor sleep (Pengo *et al.*, 2018; Cherpak & Van Lare, 2019; Haufe & Leeners, 2023). An increase in progesterone may also decrease levels of GABA in the late luteal phase, potentially causing some of the symptoms of premenstrual syndrome. As we saw in Chapter 2, GABA is a key player in sleep onset in that it helps the body to relax via suppression of the central nervous system. If GABA levels are reduced, then its relaxing properties will be less impactful. Progesterone is also a precursor of the stress hormone cortisol, which may therefore elevate cortisol levels in the luteal phase when progesterone levels are high. This has implications for melatonin concentration since cortisol suppresses serotonin, which is a precursor of melatonin (Cherpak & Van Lare, 2019). This has a resultant effect on a woman's sleep pattern since, as you may recall, melatonin is the hormone that signals to the body if it is night or day and therefore time for sleep or wake.

However, in all cases it is the *rate of change* in hormone levels that seems to be key to the disturbances in sleep, rather than the absolute levels (Cherpak & Van Lare, 2019; Xing *et al.*, 2020).

With regard to sleep architecture, the most dramatic change in sleep across the menstrual cycle is an increased EEG activity of sleep spindles in the late (post-ovulatory) luteal phase. As we have learnt, this stage of the cycle is when progesterone and oestrogen are high, compared to the follicular phase (Pengo *et al.*, 2018). Also, remember that sleep spindles indicate a sensory shutdown as an individual heads into stage 3 sleep (deep sleep), from lighter stage 2 sleep. Therefore, this increased spindle activity may objectively indicate deeper sleep in this menstrual cycle phase (Cherpak & Van Lare, 2019). It may be that the increased sleep spindle frequency has a protective effect on sleep (Cherpak & Van Lare, 2019).

Whilst objective findings may not support the sleep disturbances women experience throughout the menstrual cycle, particularly in the late luteal phase, one cannot rule out the overarching subjective reports by women of poorer sleep (Cherpak & Van Lare, 2019). Although objective data shows sleep duration and quality remain relatively stable during the different phases of the menstrual cycle, there is convincing evidence of a variation in sleep quality and quantity throughout the menstrual cycle phases, with a decline in sleep quality as a woman ages (Cherpak & Van Lare, 2019). For example, subjective sleep complaints are most common in the days preceding and during menstruation (Baker & Driver, 2007; Goldstein & Smith, 2016), and this is primarily due to one of the key physical and psychological issues during the menstrual cycle: premenstrual syndrome (PMS).

PREMENSTRUAL SYNDROME AND SLEEP

Sleep disturbances and overall poorer sleep health are associated with premenstrual symptoms and premenstrual dysphoric disorder (PMDD), a very severe form of PMS. Variables related to sleep include bedtime, sleep quality, sleep onset latency, sleep maintenance and wake time (Jehan *et al.*, 2016). There are over 200 symptoms, and sleep can help combat many of them or be disrupted because of them. They can be physical, emotional or generic, and the type of symptoms experienced, and to what degree, varies significantly from woman to woman, cycle to cycle and over time (Nowakowski *et al.*, 2013).

Three to 8 per cent of women have clinically relevant premenstrual symptoms that they perceive as distressing, affect daily function and meet clinical diagnostic criteria (Nowakowski *et al.*, 2013). Physical symptoms are numerous and are highlighted in the following list. They can be experienced along with relative extremes of pain, heavy bleeding and general malaise, all of which can be some of the key causes of poor sleep during menses. Around nine to 14 out of every 100 women can experience heavy bleeding during their period which may cause sleep issues (Informed Health, 2006). Of all the symptoms, cramps or pain are a significant factor for a woman's sleep loss during menses, with 69 per cent of women reporting pain as a cause of sleep loss (Pacheco & Callender, 2024). In such cases, finding good overnight sanitary protection is important for aiding sleep, perhaps a mattress protector too, alongside pain management techniques advised by a medical practitioner.

THE PHYSICAL SYMPTOMS OF PREMENSTRUAL SYNDROME

- Headaches
- Fatigue
- Lower back pain
- Abdominal cramps
- Nausea
- Constipation
- Diarrhoea
- Swelling or tenderness in the breasts
- Cyclic acne
- Swelling of the limbs and abdomen
- Joint or muscle pain
- Food cravings
- Changes in libido

Psychological examples of PMS tend to be increased irritability, anxiety and depression, and an overall heightened emotional sensitivity (mood swings, outbursts of anger and confusion). A broader base of psychological symptoms can also include stress, concentration difficulties, changes in appetite, moodiness, social withdrawal, tension or general unhappiness. As one may expect, the luteal phase, where premenstrual symptoms are prevalent, is also associated with the sleep disorder insomnia (the occurrence of which is more likely in women than men, particularly as they age) and a general worsening of sleep quality, given the reciprocal relationship between sleep and many of the symptoms listed as part of PMS (Nowakowski *et al.*, 2013; Pengo *et al.*, 2018; Cherpak & Van Lare, 2019; Haufe & Leeners, 2023). All these listed symptoms, and others, may result in nighttime issues such as frequent waking after sleep onset, non-restorative sleep, unpleasant dreams or even nightmares (see the information on nightmares in Chapter 6), and therefore a decreased overall sleep efficiency. Consequently, common daytime symptoms in the premenstrual week may also be experienced, such as sleepiness, fatigue, decreased alertness and an inability to concentrate: all factors that can decrease a woman's quality of life (Nowakowski *et al.*, 2013). Given the myriad of physical and psychological symptoms related to the menstrual cycle, it is little wonder that sleep is affected and that symptoms exacerbate poor sleep.

TEMPERATURE

Another common feature of sleep restriction during the menstrual cycle is night wakening due to an increased core body temperature. A client may be familiar with the problem of going to bed feeling fine, but waking in the night with sweats, a dry mouth and an overall feeling of being 'too hot' at certain points throughout their menstrual cycle. The change in core body temperature relates to the circadian rhythm I referred to in Chapter 2. The human body's core temperature has its own circadian rhythm, similar to many other body processes such as hormone release and sleep.

Before ovulation, core body temperature will elevate (by 0.3–0.6 °C) due to an increase in progesterone and, in some cases, cause an increase in wake after sleep onset, in addition to sleep fragmentation (restlessness) in the luteal phase (Cherpak & Van Lare, 2019). After ovulation, the usual rhythmic nighttime decrease in core body temperature is blunted somewhat, which is then associated with an increased wake time during the night's sleep period (Goldstein & Smith, 2016). The struggle to get to sleep through feeling hot, or waking up from feeling hot, is particularly prevalent in the luteal phase when premenstrual symptoms are rife, which can be very frustrating and affect the quality of life for a number of women. Fluctuations in REM sleep duration have also been observed as a function of nighttime body temperature during the luteal phase (Xing *et al.*, 2020). You may recall from Chapter 2 that REM sleep is associated with the regulation of emotions. Therefore, if this stage of sleep is upset in the post-ovulation luteal phase, then this parallels the phase in which we see an increase in PMS symptoms, of which many are linked to a woman's emotional state.

Overall, the impact from sleep restriction on daily life quality throughout a woman's menstrual cycle can be great. According to the National Sleep Foundation (Pacheco & Callender, 2024), one in ten women stated that sleep problems associated with their menstrual cycle interfered with daily household tasks, their occupations and relationships, and half stated they would be somewhat likely to be sad, angry or low in mood because of their daytime sleepiness. Thirty per cent of women report disturbed sleep during their menstrual cycle, whilst 23 per cent experienced worse sleep in the week prior to menstruation (luteal phase). Similarly, mood disorders are twice as likely to occur in women than in men, with a 40 per cent greater risk of insomnia in women, and overall, women are more likely to experience delayed sleep onset (Nowakowski, 2013; Pengo *et al.*, 2018; Pacheco & Callender, 2024). Good enough reasons for some sleep strategies around a woman's cycle to be put in place.

The good news is that, on the whole, most women experience their menstrual cycle with only a few of the possible symptoms and in a relatively predictable pattern, but remember, it is individualized and can vary in symptom type, duration and intensity. Age, lifestyle and overall health can also play a role in these symptom variations, making sleep and the menstrual cycle a complex and multifaceted relationship (Rugvedh, Gundreddy & Wandile, 2023). Symptoms may also change from one cycle to the next with little to any predictable pattern. Further, in addition to hormonal influences, lifestyle factors such as diet, exercise and caffeine intake can also play a significant role in sleep patterns during the menstrual cycle. The interaction of these lifestyle factors with the described hormonal fluctuations can lead to variations in sleep efficiency and subjective sleep satisfaction (Rugvedh *et al.*, 2023). It may also be that a woman is using a form of contraception which could potentially impact her menstrual cycle, and consequently sleep, either positively or negatively, so it is worth noting if this is the case.

CONTRACEPTION AND FEMALE SLEEP

The above information about a woman's menstrual cycle and sleep is based on a woman having a natural cycle without using any type of contraception. However, many women are using some form of contraception, so how does this affect their sleep, if at all? Different forms of contraceptive exist for women, such as ovulatory thermometers, barrier methods or hormone contraceptives ('the pill'), and it is of course a personal choice as to what method they use, if at all. Sleep may still be affected throughout a woman's menstrual cycle, even if they are on a form of hormonal contraceptive, but the evidence as to how and why remains inconclusive and the effect of hormonal contraceptives on sleep has not been thoroughly investigated. Nonetheless, we know natural endocrine function has a relationship with sleep, so any disruption to this will undoubtedly have an influence on an individual's sleep quality and quantity. The extent to which it does will vary from person to person. If you would like more information on women's health and hormones, then refer to the previously mentioned experts and their research groups.

It is important to note that sleep studies across the menstrual cycle (and the wider female lifespan) suffer from methodological issues (e.g. small sample size, timing of hormone measurement, different measurement techniques of sleep and oral contraceptive use). Studies often rely on subjective sleep reports of erratic sleep, which often differ from objective sleep measures of stable sleep patterns across the cycle and are vulnerable to recall or reporting bias. Similarly, studies of women can be problematic given not all women are the same and will have a variety of reproductive hormonal profiles that change across the lifespan from puberty to the menopause (Elliott-Sale *et al.*, 2021). Individual differences in patterns of sleep disturbance and variances across the menstrual cycle play a part in the findings of studies relating to sleep and the menstrual cycle. Needless to say, there is a lot more that needs to be researched in this particular area of a woman's lifespan and sleep.

Certainly, an integrated approach to sleep and the menstrual cycle is warranted if a woman is experiencing life-debilitating symptoms. Factors including nutrition, lifestyle, medications, sleep health and potentially some hormone interventions may be critical to underpinning a woman's optimal wellness (Cherpak & Van Lare, 2019). The nutrition and medical interventions are beyond the scope of this book, but there is a plethora of information in the academic literature regarding menstrual cycle, sleep and nutrition and/or medication options. Do remember that clients on the UK Anti-Doping (UKAD) testing pool need to adhere to the World Anti-Doping Association's (WADA) guidance on supplements and medication. Chapter 9 provides more information on this.

As we have seen, sleep can help combat menstrual symptoms or be disrupted because of them. That is, it has a bidirectional relationship with this phase of a woman's lifespan. Whilst there is a paucity of research on the overlap of the sleep and menstrual cycles, there is compelling evidence from which to depict how the quality and quantity of sleep may vary based on menstrual cycle phase. Most women experience the menstrual cycle with only a few predictable annoyances, but it is important to seek support where symptoms become life-affecting, particularly in relation to a woman's sleep. Where a client has sleep issues related to the menstrual cycle, encourage them to seek support where appropriate, for example, for pain management, relaxation or psychological techniques. Some tips on sleep health during the menstrual cycle are outlined below along with relevant signposting at the end of this book.

SLEEP TIPS FOR THE MENSTRUAL CYCLE

The below are specific tips relating to sleep and the menstrual cycle. For more generic sleep strategies, refer to Chapter 9.

- Pain management techniques including anti-inflammatory medication can help, but seek advice from a medical practitioner first.
- Keep a sleep diary to track menstrual cycle and sleep. Identify if sleep is affected at particular points in the cycle.
- Have water to hand overnight in case there is a need to cool down because of a rise in core body temperature, or a need to take some pain relief.
- Have a good overnight sanitary solution in case heavy flow causes night wakening.
- Have back-up nightwear/bedding ready in case there is a need to change in the night (night sweats or heavy flow). If possible, swap to another bed if uncomfortable during the night. Try not

to be awake overly long, use dim lighting and get comfortable as soon as possible.

- Sleep in comfortable and breathable clothing or naked if preferred.
- Plan ahead. If there is a likelihood of experiencing symptoms at some point in the week, be prepared.

CHAPTER 5

Female Sleep Specifics: Fertility and Pregnancy

Choosing to start, and having, a family can be a significant phase in a woman's lifespan so when considering sleep through this stage, one cannot fail to reflect on the impact of fertility and pregnancy on sleep, and vice versa. There are lots of potential sleep disturbances within these phases of a woman's lifespan, which I will describe throughout this chapter, and I will also offer some practical advice for aiding sleep during this time.

It may seem rather insensitive to discuss fertility and sleep and then follow on with pregnancy and sleep guidelines, but this is a book about the lifespan of women's sleep, so all angles will be covered. If you or your clients are particularly sensitive to these topics, then hold off until the time is right for you or your client(s) to take on board the information.

FERTILITY AND SLEEP

Before a woman finds herself at the point of being an expectant parent, there is her fertility to consider, which seems to have a reciprocal relationship with sleep and, you may not be surprised to read, is not without complexity.

The impact of sleep on fertility, or, more specifically, reproductive function, is largely unknown (Caetano *et al.*, 2021). It is a niche area of research with a lack of empirical evidence around the effects of sleep on fertility, and vice versa. The lack of research is surprising, given that sleep plays such a critical role in an individual's physical and emotional health and wellbeing: components which play a fundamental part in fertility for both men and women. Naturally, there is a role for sleep in the fertility of both men and women, but for the purposes of this book I will focus on women's fertility and sleep.

You may wonder why I have included this aspect of a woman's lifespan in this book when the evidence for the impact of sleep on it is so complex, yet scarce. However, one cannot ignore the fact that reproductive pathways may be affected through sleep restriction, and this is increasingly reported as one of the links to fertility issues in both men and women (Lateef & Akintubosun, 2020).

Whilst fertility itself is not strictly a hormone transition in the same way that puberty, pregnancy or the menopause are, there are a host of hormones involved in a woman's fertility journey to becoming a parent, and sleep plays an integral part.

Studies that evaluated the impact of sleep on hormone secretion in relation to fertility have come to different conclusions, and many are limited by small sample size, similar to studies relating to other aspects of female health and sleep. Nonetheless, throughout the literature, women with fertility issues report high rates of sleep disruption and poorer sleep quality. In fact, approximately one in three women with poor fertility report disturbed sleep and poor sleep quality (Beroukhim *et al.*, 2022). These associations are likely reciprocal, and therefore I see it as an important phase in a woman's lifespan to address.

Infertility is defined by the inability to conceive within 12 months, for women under 35 years of age, and six months for women aged 35 years or older. According to the World Health Organization, less than half (37%) of fertility problems relate to females (Goldstein & Smith, 2016), the most common cause being ovulatory dysfunction (including accompanying reproductive ageing). However, anatomical abnormalities (particularly of the fallopian tubes or uterus), endometriosis, cervical factors, medical disorders or lifestyle factors may also be responsible (Goldstein & Smith, 2016).

In considering sleep and fertility, it's important to define which aspects of sleep disturbance and reproductive capacity we are referring to. The relevant areas of *sleep disturbance* could include sleep fragmentation (restlessness), sleep continuity disturbance (broken sleep), short or long sleep duration, circadian dysrhythmia (upset daily rhythms) and/or hypoxia (a lack of oxygen). With respect to *reproductive capacity*, problems in the areas of fertility, conception, implantation, gestation, delivery and/or neonatal health could occur. However, little is known about which form of sleep disturbance is related to reproductive capacity and which specific aspects of reproductive capacity are particularly affected. The focus in this chapter will be on fertility and sleep. For a wider perspective on reproductive capacity and sleep, please refer to the academic literature and the resources and references provided at the end of this book.

Whilst the jury is still out on a direct relationship between fertility and sleep, sleep is the time when reproductive hormones are most active; they are secreted in time with the body's circadian rhythms, helping to regulate sleep patterns (Nowakowski *et al.*, 2013; Lateef & Akintubosun, 2020; Beroukhim *et al.*, 2022). Even with the limited research evidence, it can be argued that sleep has a very relevant role in attaining pregnancy. Some studies have purported a link between stress, sleep disruption and circadian misalignment, thus affecting fertility (Kloss *et al.*, 2015; Goldstein & Smith, 2016; Cherpak & Van Lare, 2019). Certainly, studies relating to irregular hours of work and pregnancy have reported that exposure to shift work or long working hours during pregnancy could be associated with the risk of adverse pregnancy outcomes. However, the results remain conflicting and inconclusive (Cai *et al.*, 2019). Nonetheless, it seems that reproductive function has an association with the body's circadian rhythm and the light–dark cycle (Lateef & Akintubosun, 2020; Beroukhim *et al.*, 2022).

Undoubtedly, some of the consequences of poor sleep may contribute to fertility issues in women. Growing evidence does suggest that sleep disruption or sleep disorders are associated with impaired reproductive function in women (Beroukhim *et al.*, 2022). However, short sleep time and impaired sleep parameters are also associated with low socioeconomic status, sedentary time and other potential confounders, making it difficult to establish whether associations between sleep and fertility are due to a causal link or associated with other issues (Beroukhim *et al.*, 2022). An additional complication is the difficulty in separating the direction of relationships among sleep, fertility and shared comorbidities such as obesity, diabetes, cardiovascular disease, mental disorders and stress. Are fertility issues and shared comorbidities responsible for troubled sleep or sleep disorders, or is it in fact the reverse (Auger, Healy-Profitós & Wei *et al.*, 2021)?

The reciprocal relationship between sleep and fertility refers to the fact that disturbed sleep may interfere with fertility processes and/or fertility issues may contribute to poor sleep quality and duration. Research has suggested that this reciprocal relationship means that sleep disturbances, and their associated consequences, may not only follow but also interfere with reproductive processes (Kloss *et al.*, 2015). The reproductive hormones oestrogen and progesterone may modify sleep, or, conversely, sleep disruption may alter the profile of reproductive hormone secretion. As levels of reproductive hormones are affected by sleep restriction, a woman's fertility is therefore affected, not only by the sleep quality but also the timing and duration of sleep (Lateef & Akintubosun, 2020). However, the relevance of these changes with regard to fertility is unclear and warrants further investigation (Goldstein and Smith, 2016).

ENDOCRINE FACTORS, FERTILITY AND SLEEP

There are some crucial endocrine players involved in fertility (and reproduction more widely), and these also have a purported interaction with sleep. Thyroid-stimulating hormone (TSH), a key hormone acting on the metabolism of almost every cell in the body, is important for reproduction. Coming from the thyroid gland, which interacts with the ovaries, the thyroid hormones are involved in almost all phases of reproduction from ovulation to formation of the placenta (Cho, 2015).[1] TSH levels increase during sleep, but sleep restriction can also be associated with higher increases in levels of TSH, which have been linked to reproductive irregularities such as anovulation (irregular periods), miscarriages and amenorrhea (when menses stops in a woman of reproductive age) (Lateef & Akintubosun, 2020). Unfortunately, many of the studies of sleep restriction and fertility have mixed methodologies, with sleep restriction displaying inconsistent effects on TSH secretion. Whilst acute, extreme sleep restriction is associated with an increase in the secretion of TSH, chronic, modest sleep restriction suppresses its secretion (Beroukhim *et al.*, 2022).

Prolactin, a hormone linked to milk production (lactation) in

---

1   The placenta is a specialized organ that plays a significant role during pregnancy. It is responsible for providing nutrition and oxygen to the foetus as well as removing waste material and carbon dioxide.

pregnancy, is also dysregulated with sleep disturbances and can be related to certain reproductive conditions, such as polycystic ovary syndrome (PCOS) and endometriosis, both associated with fertility issues (Lateef & Akintubosun, 2020). PCOS is a common condition which affects how a woman's ovaries work and causes irregular periods, excess androgen (a hormone that regulates the development and maintenance of male characteristics) and polycystic ovaries (many cysts in the ovaries). Endometriosis, as described previously, is a long-term and painful condition, where tissue similar to that of the lining of the womb grows in other places, and can play havoc with a woman's fertility. It is beyond the scope of this chapter to investigate sleep and such gynaecological conditions, but note that the psychological aspect of the pain and stress of these conditions may potentially impact a woman's sleep. More detail on pain and women's sleep is provided in Chapter 7, and further resources are available at the end of this book for areas of support if a client is living with either of these reproductive conditions.

Oestradiol, a principal hormone in puberty for development and maintenance of female sex characteristics, can be increased through sleep restriction, such as with irregular sleep routines. Oestradiol levels typically ebb and flow over the course of the menstrual cycle, and the amount of oestradiol in circulation sends messages to the hypothalamus and pituitary gland in the brain to control the development of the ovarian follicle,[2] ovulation and the menstrual cycle. Too high a level of oestradiol may upset a woman's reproductive state by interrupting ovulation.

Oestradiol is also important in reproduction as it regulates the hormones follicle-stimulating hormone (FSH) and luteinizing hormone (LH), which, as we learnt in Chapter 4, are important in the follicular phase of the menstrual cycle for ovulation and growth of the ovarian follicle. LH is specifically responsible for ovulation and development of the corpus luteum, which is the mature follicle in the ovary ready to move into the fallopian tube for potential conception – a significant stage in a woman's monthly fertile window (Lateef & Akintubosun, 2020). Shorter sleep may lead to a lower level of FSH, which may have a negative consequence for ovulation and therefore a woman's fertility (Beroukhim

---

2   The follicle is the functional unit of the ovary. It is a fluid-filled sac in the ovary containing a developing egg and plays a crucial role in the maturation and release of an egg capable of fertilization.

et al., 2022). Similarly, LH is affected by sleep restriction in that it is downregulated without sleep (Lateef & Akintubosun, 2020). Without sufficient levels of LH, ovulation will certainly be compromised.

In Chapter 2 I described the relationship between melatonin, light and sleep. Melatonin can also influence reproductive function by synchronizing sexual behaviour towards seasons and stages appropriate for mating and conception to occur (Lateef & Akintubosun, 2020). However, altered sleep patterns dysregulate the endogenous secretion of melatonin and therefore may impair reproductive health (Beroukhim *et al.*, 2022).

Melatonin also has a protective effect on the immature egg (oocyte) in that high levels of melatonin are found in the ovarian follicles, where it protects the oocyte from oxidative stress.[3] Where sleep has been compromised, lower levels of melatonin are present in the ovarian follicles, thus exposing follicles to free radicals and therefore reducing egg quality and quantity (Lateef & Akintubosun, 2020; Beroukhim *et al.*, 2022). Further, high melatonin levels have been associated with delayed puberty and impaired ovulation (Beroukhim *et al.*, 2022).

FERTILITY AND STRESS

Fertility involves a complex and highly time-sensitive process, and if the body's balance (homeostatic) mechanisms are disrupted through a lack of sleep, then these processes are thrown off-kilter and fertility issues may follow (Beroukhim *et al.*, 2022). For example, physiological stress seems to be a principal player in fertility and sleep, with sleep restriction causing higher levels of oxidative stress. This stimulates the stress response though the hypothalamic–pituitary–adrenal axis (HPA), which sends a stress signal to the body that, in evolutionary terms, the conditions for reproduction are unfavourable. The circadian dysregulation caused by the stress response (real or perceived) causes the body's homeostasis to become threatened and the HPA activates. This in turn causes a decrease in fertility as the body prepares to protect its metabolic resources against the perceived stress. This is the 'fight or flight' response and, whilst reversible, the longer a person is in a stressed state, the more likely sleep

---

3   Oxidative stress is where there is an imbalance between free radicals (toxic by-products of oxygen metabolism) and antioxidants (designed to combat the free radicals) in the body, which can cause significant damage to living cells and tissues and potentially result in certain disease states.

disturbances will prevail and the stress response continue (Cherpak & Van Lare, 2019), thus having a potential negative consequence for fertility processes. This 'stress response' has links with the psychological state of a woman too, given the bidirectional relationship sleep has with mental health (more on this in Chapter 7). Briefly, psychological stress may impact reproductive potential, and/or impaired reproductive function may worsen psychological distress. Moreover, general stress may induce or exacerbate sleep disturbance and vice versa, and both may independently or collectively impact reproduction (Beroukhim *et al.*, 2022). You can start to see how sleep and fertility have a complex relationship linked to a woman's psycho-physiological state, and whilst the interaction between psychological stress and disturbed sleep in reproduction has had limited research, it may be a crucial factor to consider during the evaluation and treatment of fertility issues (Goldstein & Smith, 2016).

IVF

An important point to consider with fertility and sleep is the influence of sleep over in vitro fertilization (IVF). This is an increasingly common method of helping a couple to have a baby and has experienced huge growth and development since the establishment of the Human Fertilisation and Embryology Authority (HEFA) in 1991, the world's first statutory regulatory body of assisted reproduction treatment and research involving the human embryo.

To put it in context, the process began in humans in the late 1970s and its use has more than doubled since 1996. According to HEFA, in 1991 there were around 6700 IVF cycles recorded at licensed fertility clinics in the UK. By 2019, the number of cycles had increased to over 69,000. Yet, despite the increased resources devoted to IVF, the procedure is still largely unsuccessful, with more than 50 per cent of cycles failing to result in live birth. Factors exacerbated by sleep restriction, including excessive stress responses, psychological distress and imbalances between free radicals and the body's antioxidant responses, are all potentially detrimental to IVF outcomes or result in a discontinuation of the IVF process.

This isn't to say poor sleep would be the sole cause of an unsuccessful IVF attempt, but sleep disturbance is recognized as the most significant psychological stressor experienced by women with fertility issues undergoing IVF. Therefore, the sleep patterns in women undergoing

IVF are an important area of research, yet available studies are limited (Beroukhim *et al.*, 2022).

Nonetheless, consistent good sleep may potentially be associated with improved IVF outcomes (Goldstein & Smith, 2016). For a more comprehensive probe into the research, do refer to some of the resources and references at the end of this book.

In summary, fertility may affect sleep and vice versa, yet the evidence as to how and to what extent sleep affects fertility in women remains scarce. Studies remain inconclusive as to a direct relationship between fertility and sleep, but undoubtedly some of the consequences of poor sleep may contribute to fertility issues in both men and women. There are contradictory findings in the literature, and the research is also limited by small sample sizes, a lack of direct comparison of reproductive health or hormones with sleep quality, and using male research samples.

Regardless, sleep is essential to human health, and when altered, it is associated with impaired reproductive function and generally poorer reproductive outcomes. It is such a complex area and the mechanisms by which sleep affects the female reproductive axis (the hypothalamic–pituitary–ovarian (HPO) axis[4]) are likely multifactorial, including factors relating to lifestyle, environment and physiological or psychological disease (Beroukhim *et al.*, 2022).

In terms of improving reproductive capacity and outcomes, sleep remains an under-investigated, adjustable concept that may provide a non-pharmacological, cost-effective and patient-centred approach. Through applying improved sleep health practices alongside psychological therapies and other interventions, the impact on a woman's fertility could be quite significant (Beroukhim *et al.*, 2022).

In relation to fertility, good sleep practices remain paramount. It's

4   The term 'hypothalamic–pituitary–ovarian (HPO) axis' refers to the collective system of female reproductive health involving the hypothalamus, pituitary gland and gonadal glands. The HPO axis releases hormones, generates female characteristics and achieves fertility.

obviously a confidential matter if a woman is trying to conceive, but if your client(s) is experiencing difficulties in conceiving and you do have a dialogue with them about it, remember to also consider their sleep. Clearly, it is not certain that good sleep will equate to successfully conceiving and a positive pregnancy outcome, but given the healthy lifestyle associations with fertility in general, it is worth discussing sleep with your client. It may also be that they are experiencing sleep issues because of the anxiety and stress that may come hand in hand with struggling to conceive, and it is here that some signposting and practical strategies may be of use.

Evidently, this is a very emotive area, so always listen to your client regarding any sleep issues relating to their fertility, signpost where necessary and, in some cases, just be their sounding board until they are ready to move forward in looking for sleep, or wider, support.

PREGNANCY, THE POSTPARTUM PHASE AND SLEEP

Hopefully, a woman has a happy and healthy relationship with her fertility and at some point(s) in her reproductive lifespan, if she so wishes, becomes pregnant. Here in this hormone transition phase, there are (once again) sleep challenges and I will highlight some of these over this next stage of the book.

I think it's important to note at this point that not all women will experience this hormone transition phase, whether through choice or, sadly, being involuntarily childless. Appropriately supporting your client in either eventuality, is of course, paramount.

Pregnancy and the postpartum phases do influence sleep disturbances in most women, and these are significant stages of a woman's lifespan in her relationship with sleep. Heartburn, cramps and pelvic pain, to name a few, are all hallmarks of sleep disturbance in pregnancy. If you were in marketing and had to sell pregnancy with the associated sleep loss, you would probably struggle to enamour your target audience!

Sleep during pregnancy and the postpartum phase is affected to various degrees (Haufe & Leeners, 2023), and although limited studies exist, specifically around sleep and the reproductive hormones, pregnancy and the postpartum period (Haufe & Leeners, 2023), this chapter will look at some of the factors that go into sleep disturbance during this time. Some practical strategies to help combat sleep disturbances will also be presented at the end of the chapter.

Throughout the three trimesters of pregnancy, sleep can be affected, either when trying to fall asleep or by being woken up. Whether a woman experiences nausea, foetal football as their unborn baby likes a kick whilst they rest or the general feelings of discomfort in the latter stages of pregnancy, all link to an accumulated sleep debt during pregnancy. Not ideal for what follows with a newborn baby, when a woman's sleep is yet again challenged as they nurse and care for their baby in the postpartum phase, all whilst also experiencing the roller coaster of postpartum emotions and hormone changes. Not forgetting, a woman may also be balancing the demands and responsibilities of other family members in this phase too. All these factors relate to sleep disturbance.

During pregnancy, there are dynamic anatomical, mechanical and physiological changes which affect a woman's sleep quality and quantity, to relative degrees, and her propensity to certain sleep disorders as she progresses through pregnancy (Pengo *et al.*, 2018). Some women may experience very little effect on their sleep for the first few months of pregnancy, and only in the latter stages, as the unborn baby has grown significantly and it becomes more uncomfortable and difficult to get to or stay asleep, do they notice a difference. However, poor sleep in the first and third trimesters is quite common due to the body's responses to pregnancy during these stages.

Anatomical changes have the potential to affect sleep duration, sleep fragmentation and breathing during sleep as the musculoskeletal system is placed under great stress as the uterus and unborn baby grow and the body prepares for delivery of the baby. Frequent mechanical symptoms can include nighttime urination (nocturia), musculoskeletal pain, uterine contractions and foetal movement. For some women, these symptoms can also bridge across the trimesters. As pregnancy progresses, more symptoms affecting sleep may manifest, such as orthopnoea (difficulty in breathing whilst lying down), heartburn, leg cramps, rhinitis (irritated inside of nose causing it to be blocked or runny) and nasal congestion. In all cases, advise clients to seek support from their healthcare provider if they are at all concerned.

After the early stages of pregnancy, the second trimester is the time to gain as much sleep as possible ahead of the typically uncomfortable third trimester. Usually, sleep quality and consistency are improved during this phase, and it is during the third trimester that sleep issues predominate, with some of the physiological and mechanical factors becoming more pronounced and sleep fragmentation (restlessness) increasing.

It is more likely that the mechanical or anatomical type of symptoms will cause sleep disruption during pregnancy rather than absolute changes in hormone levels (Pengo *et al.*, 2018; Haufe & Leeners, 2023). That said, prolactin, the hormone responsible for stimulating milk production and secretion in the postpartum phase, is associated positively with sleep in that it is thought to promote deeper sleep and correlates with high sleep efficiency, a key marker of sleep quality (Haufe & Leeners, 2023).

Sleep in pregnant women is likely to be more fragmented, whether due to increased nighttime trips to the toilet or the discomfort of a growing uterus and baby. The section 'Sleep strategy 2: Sleep extension strategies' in Chapter 9 talks about 'banking' sleep (napping), which, during pregnancy, may be beneficial to help overcome the excessive daytime sleepiness sometimes experienced by pregnant women, or help with the pending lack of sleep when due date looms. More on sleep extension strategies later in the book, but briefly, if a pregnant woman has the circumstances, opportunity and motivation to have a nap, then the general rule is to nap for 20–30 minutes and ideally between two and four o'clock in the afternoon.

Nausea and vomiting can play a large part in the disruption of a woman's sleep during pregnancy. The term 'morning sickness' is a misnomer as pregnancy-related nausea and sickness can strike at any hour of the day. The majority of pregnant women (eight out of ten) will experience some form of nausea, and for most this will improve and completely stop around 16 to 20 weeks, although for some women it can last longer. Unfortunately, some pregnant women experience extreme nausea and vomiting. They might be being sick many times in a day and be unable to keep food or drink down, which can impact on their daily life, health and, of course, their sleep. In severe cases, a woman may suffer from *hyperemesis gravidarum*, excessive nausea and vomiting that often needs hospital treatment (NHS, 2023). If this is the case for a client of yours, then they need to take advice from their GP and obstetrics team as soon as possible.

To add to the cocktail of sleep disturbances in pregnancy, a raised core body temperature, hormone fluctuations and heartburn can also manifest. With heartburn, advising your clients to avoid eating spicy food may help, and there are some over-the-counter medications a woman can try, but remind them that their GP should advise on any medications in the first instance. To prevent heartburn affecting sleep, or at least alleviate symptoms, from a practical point of view, a woman could elevate their upper body by raising the head end of the mattress or bed.

Certain sleep disorders are also common in pregnancy. Women may suffer *periodic limb movement disorder*, where an individual involuntarily moves their limbs during sleep (Haufe & Leeners, 2023), leg cramps causing waking from the pain, or *restless leg syndrome*. This is a condition where a woman may experience unpleasant sensations such as itching and an overwhelming urge to move the legs when they are at rest, particularly in the last trimester (Pengo *et al.*, 2018). Metabolic changes such as iron and folate concentrations in pregnancy are potentially more likely to increase the risk of this particular sleep disorder. In all cases, advise your client to take medical advice if they are experiencing symptoms relating to these sleep disorders.

Additionally, snoring may become an issue during pregnancy, particularly if a woman is overweight. If extreme snoring, this may be a sign of obstructive sleep apnoea (OSA), which, as described in Chapter 7, is a condition where a person's breathing is repeatedly interrupted during sleep. This can be treated clinically, so advise clients to seek medical guidance. Also, it is thought progesterone, which we know remains elevated during pregnancy, has a protective role against OSA, and it seems some pregnant women who suffer from OSA have lower levels of progesterone (Haufe and Leeners, 2023). The following list summarizes the potential symptoms in pregnancy of obstructive sleep apnoea.

POTENTIAL SYMPTOMS IN PREGNANCY OF OBSTRUCTIVE SLEEP APNOEA

- Loud snoring
- Disturbed sleep
- Morning headaches
- Sleepiness or lack of energy during daytime
- Waking up with dry mouth or sore throat
- Irritability
- Mood changes
- Loss of libido (loss of interest in sex)
- Insomnia

Short sleep duration has been shown to have an association with an increased risk of gestational diabetes, a condition where a woman without diabetes develops high blood sugar levels during pregnancy (Pengo *et al.*, 2018). All these above-mentioned conditions require intervention from an appropriately qualified clinical professional.

The position a woman sleeps in may also help with sleep quality and duration during pregnancy. This may also change with each trimester as comfort becomes more of a challenge as 'bump' develops and sleep disturbances become more prevalent. Generally, there's no harm in front sleeping until approximately 16 weeks, so long as the woman is comfortable. Even thereafter, baby is protected, but a woman probably won't be very comfortable sleeping on her front once her bump has grown to the size of a watermelon! Side sleeping on the left side is often advised when pregnant to avoid compressing major arteries, thus aiding blood flow for both mum and baby. However, there are mixed reports in the literature as to the adverse effects on pregnancy of side sleeping and indeed supine sleeping (lying on the back). Supine sleeping may compress the spine and may not be overly comfortable once a woman is into the latter stages of pregnancy (Silver *et al.*, 2019). Equally, if a woman is not normally a side sleeper, but in pregnancy tries to sleep in this position, then they may struggle to feel comfortable. Trying different ways to be comfortable is key, so bending knees whilst lying on their side, using pillows and wedges, along with a comfortable mattress or mattress topper can help. Suffice to say, as with anything sleep related, advise your pregnant clients to do what works for them to allow them to be in a safe and comfortable position to fall asleep. If they are particularly concerned about their sleeping position during pregnancy, advise them to speak to their obstetrician or midwife.

There are also the psychological aspects of pregnancy and sleep to consider too. We know that mental health has a reciprocal relationship with sleep, and it may be a woman is experiencing some mental health issues relating to pregnancy that could be affecting her sleep. Whilst pregnancy is an exciting time, it can also be a highly emotional and anxious period, which can influence sleep in terms of insomnia-like symptoms (i.e. difficulty in initiating or maintaining sleep, early waking or non-restorative, poor-quality sleep). If these symptoms are severe and continue up to three times a week, for 30 minutes or more and for over three months, then your client should speak to their GP. Signposting to some gentle psychological or relaxation techniques (see Chapter 9) or suggesting that they speak to a healthcare professional may also be useful. If you suspect a client is experiencing mental ill health, then do refer them to their GP for clinical support.

> A note on mental health for clarity. Poor mental health is a state of being that has a negative impact on the way a person thinks, feels and behaves. It can cause distress or inability in social, work or family settings and impact on daily living, including how a person relates to and interacts with those around them.
>
> Mental ill health, on the other hand, is where the degree of difficulty and length of time it has been experienced impact a person's wellbeing and functioning to the extent that it could be a diagnosable mental health condition, and it generally has a more significant detrimental impact on life (Mental Health First Aid England first aid course, 2023, personal communication).

Generally, sleep quality worsens and sleep duration is shortened as pregnancy progresses (Haufe & Leeners, 2023). For most women, managing sleep in pregnancy is straightforward, and finding general guidelines on battling some of the symptoms is relatively easy, but each pregnancy is different and highly individualized, and unfortunately, for some women, poor sleep in pregnancy can be all-consuming and the associated fatigue quite debilitating throughout the whole pregnancy. With relatively normal pregnancy-related restricted sleep, the general rule for coping is to do what works for the individual to get them through each day. Pregnancy symptoms can change hour by hour, day by day, so what works one night to help a woman sleep may not succeed on another night. Advise your clients to monitor how they're sleeping throughout their pregnancy and make changes accordingly. Sleep during this time is an absolute necessity, and women should aim to value, protect and prioritize rest and opportunities to sleep or even just to have a nap. Easier said than done, especially if a woman already has a family and they are not experiencing their first pregnancy. Naps in particular can help as pregnancy fatigue can hit like a steam roller at any time, so advising women to use opportunities to get good sleep when they can is useful, but remain pragmatic. Also, a certain amount of self-awareness and finding their own way through their pregnancy means a woman can feel in control (to a certain degree), at a time when they are experiencing invasion of the body snatchers. Boring as it sounds, early nights will become a sanctuary, and they shouldn't beat themselves up about missing the monthly drinks date if not feeling up to it and prioritizing their sleep.

Once a woman has her baby, there is a whole new way of life to contend with, and exciting and incredible as it is, it does bring more sleep challenges. Post-pregnancy sleep is different for every woman, but for certain, there will be relatively little of it for any woman, no matter how much help and support they have.

POSTPARTUM SLEEP

'Postpartum' refers to the hazy period in a woman's life, immediately post childbirth and up to six months post birth. It typically involves three continuous phases: acute, subacute and delayed. The acute phase lasts for six to 12 hours post birth, subacute for six weeks, and the delayed phase up to six months. It is often defined as the period of time after delivery of the baby when maternal physiological and anatomical changes return to the non-pregnant state. During this phase, a woman's sleep will undoubtedly be disturbed, quite significantly in some cases, although this is a less well-understood area than some of the other areas of female sleep health (Nowakowski et al., 2013).

Hormone changes are rife during the postpartum phase, and with regard to sleep, this can be an issue. If the woman is not breastfeeding, oestrogen and progestogen levels tend to decline quite quickly after the birth, usually returning to regular menstrual function by the sixth to eighth week postpartum.

However, if the woman is breastfeeding, then oxytocin[5] and prolactin[6] hormone levels predominate, and the menstrual cycle is supressed by the frequency and intensity of breastfeeding. Breastfeeding means high levels of prolactin, which inhibit the ovarian response to follicle-stimulating hormone, which in turn suppresses the release of luteinizing hormone, the key hormone in ovulation (Chauhan & Tadi, 2024). Melatonin levels may also be altered in the postpartum phase, resulting in higher concentrations of melatonin upon wakening, suggesting a

---

5   Oxytocin is a principal hormone for breastfeeding. Its main role is to ensure the ejection of milk through the breasts when the baby sucks and to trigger the mechanisms necessary to sustain the supply throughout breastfeeding.
6   Prolactin stimulates milk production for breastfeeding.

'phase shift' of the circadian rhythm in postpartum women. This refers to the fact that bedtime and wake-up time will move to either earlier in the day (phase advance) or later in the day (phase delay), which has a consequential effect on sleep patterns and other daily rhythms (Thomas & Burr, 2006). Remember from the description of sleep regulation in Chapter 2 that melatonin levels need to be high to signal sleep, and if they are lowered overnight, then sleep may be restricted somewhat.

Increases in sleep difficulties are observed not only through the quite acute hormonal drop of oestrogen and progesterone following delivery of the baby, but also through specific characteristics of the postpartum period, such as the unpredictable sleeping rhythms of the infant or their need to feed during the night (Haufe & Leeners, 2023; Nowakowski, 2013).

Whether it is the first, second or third time round (or more!), the demands on a woman's sleep when she has a newborn can be quite significant, with increased levels of wake after sleep onset and a decrease in sleep efficiency compared to other times during pregnancy (Nowakowski *et al.*, 2013). The good news is that sleep tends to normalize from approximately three to six months postpartum as, typically, this is when an infant's sleep will start to regulate as they recognize the difference between night and day. However, a woman's fatigue levels can remain high up until the first year after delivery (Nowakowski *et al.*, 2013), though this very much depends on the woman's circumstances and baby.

Many factors need to be considered in relation to a woman's sleep and the postpartum phase, aside from the hormonal influence on sleep. To name a few, a woman's age, type of delivery, method of infant feeding and the baby's temperament, along with a possible return to work, other family responsibilities and availability of nighttime support, can all impact on a women's sleep quality and quantity during the postpartum phase (Nowakowski *et al.*, 2013).

Do be aware that approaching sleep discussions with mums of newborns can be a sensitive topic. For your clients, now is not the time to advise them to sleep when the baby sleeps. Whilst this may seem like good advice, it can sound quite patronizing (so I've been told by audiences of new mums!) and it's not very practical. Yes, if a woman has the circumstances, opportunity and motivation to grab a nap when their baby is sleeping, then do so. However, be aware that believing they *must* sleep in the daytime when the baby is asleep can often be a source of stress for a mum, especially if they have other responsibilities, such as other young children at home. For some women, this is a time to get other aspects of their day complete, whether that is having a shower, doing some light exercise, spending time with other family members or catching up on some work (or all of the above!). Any of these can have a positive effect on a postpartum mum's state of mind and therefore later sleep quality. So refrain from suggesting naps are for all when there may be other activities that may help a postpartum mum get some good nighttime sleep. Of course, there definitely is a time to be 'pulling up the drawbridge' and snuggling in with a newborn when a woman can, but also encourage them to be pragmatic; life can be hectic, and each woman should deal with their postpartum sleep as best they can.

One aspect to be aware of with clients in the postpartum phase is postpartum depression (PPD), one of the most common complications among postpartum women. Women with higher levels of fatigue, poor sleep quality and low resilience levels are at a higher risk of developing PPD (Baattalia *et al.*, 2023). It is beyond the scope of this chapter to go into detail around PPD, but as healthcare providers, be aware of this condition and refer to medical support where necessary. Signposting for postpartum support is available at the end of this book, and more details of mental health conditions associated with pregnancy or the postpartum period are available in Chapter 7.

Below are some sleep tips to help during a woman's pregnancy and postpartum phase. If a woman is living with some of the sleep disturbances highlighted in this chapter, then refer them to their obstetric team or GP for support. (For more generic sleep strategies, refer to Chapter 9.)

SLEEP TIPS FOR PREGNANCY

- Ensure good hydration, ideally 6–8 glasses of fluid per day.
- If leg cramps cause wakening, breathe slowly through the pain; it will pass. Have a drink of water and try to get back to sleep as soon as possible.
- Sleep in loose-fitting, breathable clothing.
- Sleep in a comfortable position and have lots of supportive pillows, particularly in the third trimester.

- Try side sleeping with knees and hips bent or using pillows to alleviate lower back pressure. Check with a GP or midwife for correct sleeping positions during pregnancy.
- Accept the need to urinate more, especially at night and in the third trimester. Minimize it through drinking less in the hour before bedtime.
- Eat bland foods to try to avoid heartburn. If heartburn becomes a problem at night, sleep with the head elevated on pillows.
- Where possible, catch up on lost sleep through sleep extension techniques such as napping.
- Try to get some relaxation time during the day to help with any aches and pains or psychological stressors. This will help with getting to sleep or having a daytime nap. Check with the midwife or obstetric team that the chosen relaxation technique is safe.
- Rest as much as possible ahead of the birth, after which sleep will undoubtedly be compromised.

CHAPTER 6

Female Sleep Specifics: Perimenopause and Menopause

Without doubt, I am regularly asked in my work as a sleep health practitioner about the effects of perimenopause and menopause on sleep and how to combat them. The simple answer is yes, sleep and the menopause transition do have a relationship, but how a woman will cope and respond to the many possible symptoms during this phase, in particular poor sleep, is entirely individualized. Nevertheless, there are some generic methods to relieve symptoms and their effect on sleep in this phase of a woman's lifespan. I'll describe these methods throughout this chapter along with a description of some of the sleep disturbances and their effects.

WHAT IS THE MENOPAUSE?

Every woman goes through the menopause, a normal and expected phase in a woman's lifetime. It is a natural event, typically due to age and defined as the stage in a woman's lifespan when their periods stop completely (12 months without any menstrual bleeds), ovaries end their monthly cycle of producing the ovarian hormones oestrogen and progesterone, and pregnancy cannot occur naturally.

Definitions of the terms 'perimenopause' and 'menopause' can vary, with menopause commonly used to mean both the transition period as a whole and the point when menses has finally ceased happening. 'Perimenopause' is used to describe a varying duration of time between when menstrual cycles begin to change and the point at which menses ceases (Bazeley, Marren & Shepherd, 2022). Basically, it is the phase leading into the menopause. The perimenopause typically starts in a woman's forties, but can show signs in her thirties, or even earlier. Following on from this phase, usually, in a healthy woman, menopause occurs in their early fifties. Here in the UK, menopause happens at approximately 52 years of age, but in some circumstances it can be earlier due to impaired ovarian function or certain medical interventions such as chemotherapy (Nowakowski, 2021). Either way, the effects of the menopause on a women's quality of life are far-reaching and go beyond a biological midlife change.

The time frames of the perimenopause and menopause mean the entire process of the menopause transition may have to be endured by a woman for anywhere from two to ten years, sometimes longer. Combined with this is the fact that the impact of menopause can linger for some years after the event. Therefore, a woman's perimenopausal and menopausal state can potentially last for up to a third of her life and, consequently, given the longevity of the menopause transition process, the possible effects of this phase on sleep can be chronic and debilitating. Therefore, it should not be underestimated how much the menopause transition is a significant chapter in a woman's lifespan, culminating in the end of a biological function. Yet it is not a subtle event that occurs at a precise moment in time; it is a shift in a woman's biology over several years (Hill, 1996). For brevity, I'll use 'menopause' as a generic term throughout the remainder of this chapter to describe this stage of a woman's lifespan, encompassing both the perimenopause and menopause itself.

In the UK, it is estimated that 13 million women are currently going through or have experienced the menopause (Houses of Parliament Committee, 2021; Bowling, 2023). Worldwide, the population of menopausal and postmenopausal women is projected to increase to 1.2 billion by 2030 (Hill, 1996). Therefore, it is a priority for clinical settings, industry and wider society that any impacts on health through this phase of a woman's life are highlighted and addressed with regard to support available, information and education. Clearly, any number of years is a significant amount of time for a woman to be experiencing the symptoms of the menopause (outlined below), and it is important that awareness and education around this phase of a woman's life are highlighted. This chapter will play a small part in addressing the issues around sleep and the menopause.

MENOPAUSE SYMPTOMS

It is the erratic changes in hormone levels of oestrogen and progesterone that cause menopause symptoms, of which there are several. Similar to the menstrual cycle and pregnancy, unpredictable hormone levels can be extremely hard to manage, and the perimenopause phase, in particular, is troublesome as the ovaries are really in a state of flux and will keep a woman guessing from month to month, or day to day, how they will behave in terms of hormone secretion. It is little wonder that some women describe this phase as being terribly complicated in trying to balance their own health, work demands, family responsibilities and keeping on top of the daily juggle. Managing all these factors whilst not feeling themselves due to the symptomology of this significant phase in a women's lifespan can be extremely hard for women. The maxim of 'juggling the juggle' can become all too familiar for women during this phase of their life. According to a 2022 survey by the Fawcett Society,[1] the largest survey of menopausal women conducted in the UK thus far, 77 per cent of women experience one or more menopause symptoms that they would describe as 'very difficult'.

> Of the many symptoms during the menopause, common ones include hot flushes and night sweats (vasomotor symptoms), brain fog, mood swings, anxiety, irritability, weight gain, headaches, hair loss, urinary incontinence, loss of libido and vaginal dryness. Most of these can interrupt sleep patterns and affect the quality of life for a significant portion of women of menopausal age.

An overarching symptom, and one of the most common complaints during a woman's menopause, is sleep disturbance. Sleep changes in the menopause usually manifest at first as sleep fragmentation (restlessness), increased night wakings and an overall poor sleep quality. Declining levels of oestrogen are associated with menopausal sleep disruption, but vasomotor symptoms (VMS) (hot flushes), generic age-related changes such as an increase in nocturnal urination, stress, sleep disorders (such as restless leg syndrome and breathing disorders), increases in comorbid

---

1   The Fawcett Society is a UK charity campaigning for gender equality and women's rights at work, at home and in public life.

conditions (such as depression), and use of prescription sleeping aids are also factors in the complex aetiology (Pengo *et al.*, 2018; Nowakowski, 2021; Schaedel *et al.*, 2021; Tandon *et al.*, 2022). As time goes on during the menopause, or even post-menopause, there can potentially be an increase in the sleep disorder insomnia (Nowakowski, 2021; Tandon *et al.*, 2022) which, as Chapter 7 describes in more detail, is a leading global cause of poor sleep, particularly for women.

Similar to the other areas of women's health I have described in this book, subjective and objective data on female sleep during the menopause years is not overly researched and there are some discrepancies in the findings. Some studies even report improved sleep in women of perimenopausal age. Nonetheless, the overwhelming subjective reports of poor sleep cannot be ignored. Figure 6.1 illustrates the Catch-22 situation which can exist with sleep and menopause symptoms to the point where some women's quality of life is severely affected. Some women unfortunately cannot get out of the spiral of a lack of sleep causing a worsening of menopause symptoms, which then leads to poorer sleep and an increase in menopause symptomology. This is a positive feedback loop which perpetuates unless a successful intervention is found.

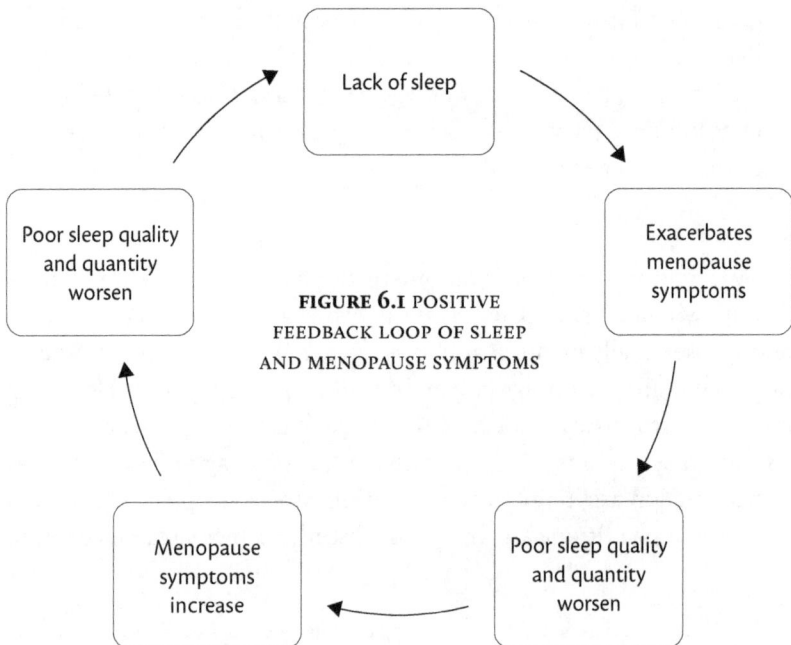

FIGURE **6.1** POSITIVE FEEDBACK LOOP OF SLEEP AND MENOPAUSE SYMPTOMS

The Fawcett Society's report (2022) stated that the menopause symptoms most often described in their survey as 'very or somewhat difficult' were difficulty sleeping (84%) and poor memory or concentration or difficulty focusing on tasks, sometimes called 'brain fog' (73%). Similarly, the Menopause Mandate survey (2024) reported that 70 per cent of women cited brain fog, fatigue and low mood as menopause symptoms.

From a mental health point of view, 69 per cent of women surveyed in the Fawcett Society report revealed difficulties with anxiety or depression due to menopause, and a Generation M report (GenM 2020) found that 41 per cent of menopausal women felt 'lonely, invisible, irrelevant and dispensable'. These are awful symptoms for women to be experiencing and highlight the need for more awareness and support in the area.

HORMONE CHANGES AND SLEEP IN THE MENOPAUSE

Hormone changes have been linked to poor sleep in menopause-aged women. Although poorly understood, sleep regulation seems to be directly affected by the body's supply of oestrogen. The change in hormone levels leading to lowered oestrogen levels has been associated with a lower sleep efficiency (Murphy & Campbell, 2007) and sleep-disordered breathing (Netzer, Eliasson & Strohl, 2003), whereas higher oestrogen levels have been associated with fewer night wakenings and early morning awakenings (Woods & Mitchell, 2010). Notably, it seems to be the relative *change* in oestrogen levels that causes the issues with sleep during the menopause, rather than the absolute levels themselves (Haufe & Leeners, 2023). Regardless, oestrogen has a positive association with sleep, so declining levels may cause sleep difficulties for some women and, as ever, it is an individualized response as to how much a woman is affected.

Similarly, the usual regular 24-hour rhythmicity of both follicle-stimulating hormone and luteinizing hormone during the follicular and luteal phase of the menstrual cycle sees declining levels during the menopause. Again, it is the speed of the rate of change in levels of follicle-stimulating hormone that can potentially affect sleep in menopausal women (Beroukhim *et al.*, 2022).

Lowered levels of progesterone have been associated with sleep-disordered breathing during the menopause, similar to the menstrual cycle's luteal phase when progesterone levels decline, and the proposed protective effects of progesterone on breathing reduce (it acts as a stimulant to respiration) (Netzer *et al.*, 2003). Lower progesterone levels have also been associated with increased frequency of sleep disturbances and insomnia during the menopause phase (Hatcher *et al.*, 2020).

However, it's not just ovarian hormone changes in menopause that can affect sleep. The nighttime hormone melatonin, which we talked about in Chapter 2, generally decreases its secretion with age, but also decreases specifically in relation to the menopausal state (Pengo *et al.*, 2018). So sleep regulation, the very signalling of when to sleep or wake up, is disrupted during this phase of a woman's life.

In terms of sleep architecture, stage 3 sleep (deep, slow-wave sleep) can decline in the menopause phase. Approximately 40 per cent of deep sleep is disrupted in this phase of a woman's life, and this is most likely linked to the decline in oestrogen during this time. However, higher incidences of stage 3 sleep have been reported in some women of menopausal age, which is perhaps a compensatory mechanism for the increases in sleep fragmentation and wake after sleep onset during this phase of a woman's life (Pengo *et al.*, 2018).

Post menopause, the fall in oestrogen and progesterone means that approximately 40 to 50 per cent of women will continue to experience sleep issues, whether that be sleep onset or sleep maintenance (getting to sleep or staying asleep) (Walker, 2024a). This is an estimate, and the likelihood of the problem is sadly probably greater.

VASOMOTOR SYMPTOMS

A further significant symptom of the menopause is hot flushes or, more specifically, vasomotor symptoms. Approximately 75 per cent of women suffer from vasomotor symptoms during the menopause, and they play a major role in sleep disturbances in these women. In their survey of menopausal women, the Fawcett Society (2022) listed hot flushes as the next most common problematic symptom (70%), after difficulty sleeping and 'brain fog'.

The presence of vasomotor symptoms accounts for a significant proportion of the total time awake during the night in menopausal women, although their severity does vary from woman to woman. Symptoms are associated with sleep disturbances such as sleep fragmentation (restlessness), increased wake after sleep onset, poor sleep efficiency and chronic insomnia. If we consider that the perimenopause can last anywhere from a woman's early forties to mid-fifties, then that is a significant portion of a woman's life to be experiencing the sleep-debilitating effects of hot flushes.

So what are hot flushes exactly? It seems hormones are again to blame! Hot flushes originate from the fall in oestrogen during the perimenopause phase of a woman's life. The theory is that the decrease in oestrogen somehow confuses the brain into thinking the body is overheating. It is not definitively known why this happens. This *perception* of overheating causes a cascade of physiological reactions as the body believes it needs to cool itself and quickly too. To rid itself of the *perceived* excess heat, the brain tells the body to launch a fairly aggressive *vasomotor response* (a change in blood flow); the blood vessels widen (dilate), heart rate rises, blood flow to the skin increases, and sweat glands are stimulated, causing a woman to feel hot, flushed and sweaty. These are unpleasant sensations and there is significant variability between individuals (Moe, 2004).

The vasomotor response can last anywhere from two to four minutes, or in extreme cases up to 20 minutes, which is a significant portion of time to be feeling uncomfortable, particularly at night when sleep is disrupted as a result. Equally, the subjective intensity of the vasomotor event can vary quite dramatically, ranging from 'severely disruptive' to 'mild'. The timing and duration of the hot flush is also related to the severity, and it is the *duration* of a vasomotor event, rather than the number of events during the night, that correlates with sleep fragmentation and the lighter stages of sleep experienced during a night of vasomotor symptoms (Moe, 2004). Therefore, a woman could have many hot flushes throughout the night, but of very short duration, and not be overly aware, or she could experience fewer vasomotor events, but of longer duration, and experience many interruptions to their sleep as a consequence.

Objective sleep measurements confirm that sleep variables such as *fragmentation* (restlessness), increased wake after sleep onset and poor sleep efficiency are associated with vasomotor symptoms. There is a school of thought that vasomotor activity may be dependent on the sleep stage a woman is experiencing (NREM or REM sleep) and occurs mainly in the first half of the night. Studies have found that this time in the night is when the occurrence of objectively determined vasomotor events correlated with subjective sleep complaints, such as increased night wakening (Pengo *et al.*, 2018).

Treatment options for vasomotor symptoms vary and some are outlined below. Whatever the choices available, remedies should be designed for each woman. The good news is, for most women, vasomotor symptoms spontaneously resolve in three to five years (Shen & Stearns, 2009).

MENOPAUSE AND SLEEP TREATMENT

Fortunately, hormone replacement therapy (HRT)[2] and non-hormonal therapies have been shown to improve subjective sleep quality (de Zambotti, 2014; Pengo *et al.*, 2018; Haufe & Leeners, 2023). With regard to HRT, a woman should gather information from a specialist menopause doctor with regard to her treatment options (see the resources section at the end of this book), but there are encouraging associations between HRT and sleep quality in women.

As a non-hormonal therapy option, in the recently updated National Institute for Health Care and Excellence (NICE) 2024 guidelines for menopause diagnosis and management, cognitive behavioural therapy (CBT) was mentioned as a worthy alternative treatment for some of the symptoms of menopause. NICE reported that CBT had been found to reduce the frequency and severity of hot flushes and night sweats, and should be considered alongside, or as an alternative to, hormone replacement therapy (NICE, 2024). It was also found to help sleep problems related to menopause, including how long it takes to fall asleep and how long before the person wakes. Cognitive behavioural therapy for insomnia (CBT-I) is already known to have a positive effect on insomnia (Pengo *et al.*, 2018), so the wider acknowledgment by NICE for CBT having a helpful outcome on some of the other symptoms of the menopause is a step in the right direction for women and their non-hormonal treatment options during this phase of their lifespan.

In addition to CBT, more and more frequently, industry brands are developing products to help women who experience nighttime

---

2   Hormone replacement therapy replenishes women with the ovarian hormones lost during the menopausal transition to alleviate associated symptoms. Before being prescribed HRT, women should discuss their menopause symptoms with a menopause specialist medical practitioner.

hot flushes to get a better night's sleep. For example, improved quality breathable bed linen and cooling aids in pillows are now widely available. Additionally, nutrition advice has tended to favour foods containing soy to alleviate hot flush symptomology (Nagata *et al.*, 1999) and advised against ingesting hot, spicy foods, caffeine and alcohol (Sturdee, 2008). Nutrition and sleep is a vast topic and there is some more information on this provided in Chapter 9, where I look into sleep strategies.

POST-MENOPAUSE

Some of the sleep problems experienced during the menopause can remain post menopause, and there are various explanations about what is actually causing the poor sleep quality in postmenopausal women. Is the sleep restriction these women are experiencing due to the change in hormone levels, rather than the onset of a sleep disorder (e.g. sleep apnoea or periodic limb movement) or, more simply, the general onset of ageing (Krystal *et al.*, 1998)? Certainly, postmenopausal women are more likely to be reported as having difficulty with the onset of sleep and having possible sleep onset insomnia, and are more likely to screen positive for obstructive sleep apnoea in comparison to premenopausal women (Tandon *et al.*, 2022). However, it is difficult to decipher a definitive reason for poor sleep in this demographic since women in this phase of life are typically a problematic group to study because of the likelihood of coexisting health conditions and fluctuating hormones.

MENOPAUSE NIGHTMARES

Nightmares during the menopause phase is an area I get asked about frequently. It seems to be a common symptom, if less well reported compared to, for example, hot flushes or anxiety.

There are limited studies attempting to identify risk factors for nightmares in the general population. Generally, lower socioeconomic status, insomnia, impaired sleep quality and some personality traits have been associated with nightmares, but nothing specifically on the menopause transition (Park *et al.*, 2021).

Typically occurring in the REM phase of sleep (stage 4 sleep), a nightmare is defined as an extended, extremely unhappy dream that usually involves efforts to avoid threats to survival, security or physical integrity (Cappadona *et al.*, 2021).

Symptoms of nightmares vary, but usually involve some sort of physical symptom, such as sweating and shortness of breath. They are highly emotional, with fear, anger, shame and sadness also being reported. They can occur nightly in extreme cases (nightmare disorder) or as infrequently as less than once a month.

More prevalent in women than men, nightmares are usually associated with several factors already linked with the menopause, such as sleep disruptions and insomnia, difficulties in sleep onset and maintenance, tiredness upon getting up, daytime sleepiness, lack of energy, difficulties in concentrating, and mental health issues including anxiety and depression (Cappadona *et al.*, 2021).

Nightmares can be classified as post-traumatic (direct reproduction of a traumatic event) or idiopathic (more imaginative stories, not necessarily reflecting a previous traumatic event (Cappadona *et al.*, 2021). Impaired sleep following a nightmare could also be linked to the higher autonomic (involuntary) response the body experiences as a result of a stressor such as anxiety.

Nightmare disorder is more serious and defined as the repeated occurrence of nightmares that cause clinically significant distress or impairment in social, occupational or other important areas of functioning. It is not caused by the physiological effects of drug abuse or medication, or a coexisting mental and medical disorder (Cappadona *et al.*, 2021).

The decrease in oestrogen and progesterone during the menopause can cause less deep sleep and more REM (dream) sleep, but it may not be the causative factor for women experiencing nightmares during the menopause. More likely, during this phase, any nightmares experienced are linked to the psychological state of the individual rather than the hormone transition of menopause itself. If you know a client is experiencing vivid dreams or nightmares that are causing an issue with their quality of life, then do refer them on for support from a suitable medical professional.

MENOPAUSE AND THE WORKPLACE

Women of menopausal age are the fastest-growing demographic in the UK workforce and are staying in work for longer than ever before. One in eight of the UK's workforce are women over 50, with this number rising. Yet these experienced and skilled role models often receive little support with menopause symptoms. Many women still feel there is a stigma surrounding talking about menopause and often try to hide their symptoms at work. As a result, some cut back their hours or responsibilities. Sadly, others leave work altogether, citing lower productivity, reduced work satisfaction and difficulties with time management in relation to the menopause transition as key reasons (Brewis *et al.*, 2017; Henpicked, 2021; UK Parliament, 2022). Staggeringly, the UK loses approximately 900,000 women a year from its workforce due to menopause-related issues. That's roughly the equivalent to the population of a large UK city. Yet still the menopause transition remains a taboo subject in contemporary society.

The headlines from the Fawcett Society's report on menopause (2022), which researched women's experiences of menopause in the workplace, were quite astonishing. One in ten women who have worked during the menopause have left employment due to their symptoms, with 61 per cent reporting a loss of motivation at work thanks to their symptoms, and 52 per cent citing a loss of confidence in the workplace.

Despite these figures, eight out of ten women say their employer hadn't shared information, trained staff or put in place a menopause absence policy. Almost half of women haven't approached their GPs about the menopause and three in ten of those who have done so have unfortunately experienced delays in diagnosis. Only four in ten women who have talked to their GP about the menopause say they were immediately offered hormone replacement therapy (Bazeley *et al.*, 2022). Whilst this may not be a treatment option for everyone, to not even be offered it as a possible intervention is worrying, particularly when you consider it can potentially have a positive association with a woman's sleep.

In 2023, the UK government turned down a proposal by their Women and Equalities Committee for a pilot project around menopause leave, deeming it 'counterproductive', and dismissed a recommendation to make menopause a protected characteristic under the Equality Act (BBC News, 2023). Whilst the UK government is encouraging more employers to give greater consideration to female health and the wellbeing of their employees, particularly those in the menopause, it is a sad situation if the government doesn't engage wholly with the recommendations of the Woman and Equalities Committee. That said, at the time of writing, the UK government are attempting to address female health overall through the Women's Health Strategy, with priority being given to menstrual problems and menopause, among other areas. As part of this strategy, the cost of HRT has been drastically reduced in recent years, hopefully making it more accessible for many more women. But there is still more to be done.

Times are changing, which is the good news. More and more menopause groups have been established, campaigning for better rights for woman and more education, equality and awareness around the menopause topic and its effects on a woman's ability to be 'well' in daily life during this phase of her lifespan. There is now more dialogue about menopause in the workplace and more advice is readily available for employers and employees to help navigate support for working women in this stage of their lives. For example, employers need to be aware that they should act in a fair and reasonable way to protect the health, safety and wellbeing of their employees whilst they're at work and be mindful of key legislation such as the Equality Act 2010, which protects against discrimination, and the Health and Safety at Work etc. Act 1974, which protects health and safety.

Whilst the topic of menopause in the workplace branches out of the specific issue of sleep and menopause, it highlights the impact of menopause on women in the workplace (and wider society). It is imperative that changes are made to harness the skills, experience and talents of menopausal women in order that productivity in the workplace isn't impacted further (Bazeley *et al.*, 2022). If you consider that UK industry loses billions of pounds annually due to sleep-related issues (Hafner *et al.*, 2017), it makes sense to address any concerns employees may be having in relation to sleep, menopause being one of those issues. Reform is needed in the context of support, education and information for employers, employees and medical practitioners. More information about women in the workplace and menopause is signposted at the end of this book.

MENOPAUSE SUPPORT GROUPS AND ORGANIZATIONS

A significant support group is the Menopause Mandate, established in 2022. This is a group of women who 'share a common interest in perimenopause and menopause' and are focused on 'creating a coalition of campaigners to achieve everyone's ultimate goal of revolutionizing the support and advice women receive from both our health service and wider society' in relation to the menopause.[3]

According to the Menopause Mandate 2024 survey of over 2000 women, a staggering 96 per cent reported that menopause symptoms affected their quality of life. Half took over a year to realize they might be perimenopausal or menopausal, furthering the argument for education on the topic in wider society.

Further, Generation M, who look to educate brands, retailers, employers and support networks about the menopause, reported in The GenM Invisibility Report (GenM, 2020) that three out of four women think the menopause remains a taboo subject, not talked about openly enough in society, and that 87 per cent of those experiencing the menopause thought that midlife women were overlooked by society and brands.

In the UK, there is the Menopause Charity, whose mission it is to help people understand the mental and physical changes that occur during the menopause and provide them with the tools and treatments needed to manage those. Specifically for UK healthcare providers, there is also the British Menopause Society, a specialist authority for menopause and post-reproductive health. They aim to educate, inform and guide healthcare professionals on menopause and all aspects of post-reproductive health.

Worldwide, there is the International Menopause Society (IMS), which brings together the world's leading experts to collaborate and share knowledge about all aspects of ageing in women. Their mission is to work globally to promote and support access to best-practice healthcare for women through their menopause transition and post-reproductive years, enabling them to achieve optimal health and wellbeing (International Menopause Society, 2024). They provide information not just for healthcare professionals, but for women in the general public too.

For women seeking medical help, if you have a client who is in a position to access medical input privately, then there are several UK-based specialist menopause centres that offer very good support, education and resources to this demographic. I'd encourage you and your clients to

---

3   www.menopausemandate.com

look up Dr Clare Spencer at My Menopause Centre. Dr Spencer is a very knowledgeable GP in the subject of female health, particularly perimenopause and menopause; details of My Menopause Centre are included in the resources section at the end of this book. Of course, there are also the traditional routes of support available in the UK through the National Health Service, and other support routes are also available and are signposted at the end of this book.

Parallel to the rise in menopause support groups, there is also female technology, or 'femtech', as a globally developing brand. Like or loathe the term (do we have 'mentech'?!), it refers to technology products, applications and hardware which are 'consumer-centric' and address women's health and wellbeing issues; innovation here is on the increase. Part of this is a move towards more technological support for menopausal women. For example, various smartphone applications have been developed which, using artificial intelligence (AI),[4] can help build a 'menopause profile' of the individual user and support access to information and resources during this significant phase of a woman's lifespan. The applications available can offer new capabilities to help women be better informed and have greater control of their own reproductive health, including, for example, educational content, treatment options and, crucially, tracking to identify and manage symptoms. One UK-based company claim to be able to build a profile of an individual woman from certain biological markers and by asking questions around cognitive and emotional wellbeing. This information would be used to modify the ingredients that would be then 3D-printed into supplement pills as part of a subscription-based package to support the woman's individual menopause symptoms (Mahaila, 2023). I'm not so sure about reducing human interactions for helping women achieve better health, but the concept of tailoring data intelligence around a women's personal health requirements is interesting.

SLEEP STRATEGIES IN THE MENOPAUSE

Many menopause sleep strategies are generic and can be applied to improve sleep health in any circumstances (outside of a sleep disorder).

---

4   Artificial intelligence (AI) is 'the ability of a digital computer or computer-controlled robot to perform tasks commonly associated with intelligent beings. The term is frequently applied to the project of developing systems endowed with the intellectual processes characteristic of humans, such as the ability to reason, discover meaning, generalize, or learn from past experience' (Copeland, 2024).

However, there are some sleep health strategies that are more specific to the menopause phase and are outlined below. You may already know of a client struggling with their sleep in this stage of her life, or perhaps this chapter has highlighted a conversation to have with, or at least a question to ask, a client regarding her sleep which may help you to provide more insightful support.

SLEEP TIPS FOR THE MENOPAUSE

These are specific tips relating to sleep and the menopause. For more generic sleep strategies, refer to Chapter 9.

- Wear breathable light clothing to bed, such as light cotton pyjamas, and consider keeping an extra set near the bed.
- Assess the sleep system: bed, pillow, mattress, duvet. Is it comfortable? Are the materials too light/too heavy (e.g. duvet tog)? Consider whether you can change the sleep system according to the seasons/symptom severity.
- Use a fan or air conditioning to cool the room temperature. Ideally, have the room temperature at 18–20°C before sleep.
- Have a cool bag by the bed with ice packs, cold drink, ice cubes and a cold flannel to help with night sweats.
- Try lying on a cool floor to reduce temperature. Keep lights dim and be awake for as short a time as possible. Return to bed to sleep.
- Eat healthily. Avoid large meals, especially before bedtime. Some foods that are spicy or acidic may trigger hot flushes. Try foods rich in soy as they might minimize hot flushes (check with your healthcare provider if you have a family history of breast cancer).
- Maintain a consistent, healthy weight.
- Avoid stimulants such as nicotine, caffeine and alcohol, especially before bedtime.
- Accept that the menopause is a natural process for most women and you can manage the symptoms.
- Consider seeking medical guidance on hormone replacement therapy if your symptoms are particularly life-affecting.

Hopefully, you now have some answers and solutions to female health matters and sleep. Advise on effective sleep strategies as often as you can, as the key to good sleep is *routine* and an awareness of how life and, in particular, physical or emotional factors are affecting sleep. Managing the change in hormones through the menopause will help combat some of the symptoms, and remember, every woman will respond differently, albeit subtly. Making good lifestyle choices around exercise, sleep and nutrition will undoubtedly help to navigate this phase of a woman's life. In extreme cases, where daily quality of life is being affected to a large degree, and some of the suggested practical sleep strategies aren't having the desired outcome, it may be useful to seek advice from a medical practitioner regarding more clinical interventions.

As we have seen, sleep across a woman's lifespan is compromised in many areas, not least the hormone transition phases we have just learnt about. Certainly, each phase of a woman's life, from puberty to postmenopause, increases the risk of sleep disturbance in unique ways. Given the longevity of some of the phases where a woman's sleep may be affected, it is important to consider female sleep and possible interventions to aid it. The good news is that sleep and sleep disturbances are increasingly being acknowledged as principal determinants of women's health (Kloss *et al.* 2015). Fortunately, interventions, education and support are better than ever before, but there is still more to be done.

The next few chapters will focus on some of the other areas of a woman's lifespan in which sleep may be affected where this is not necessarily directly due to hormone transitions – areas such as mental health, sleep disorders, shift work and carer responsibilities. It may be that your clients don't have sleep issues related to any of these areas, but they can be significant factors in a woman's relationship with sleep, so are worth highlighting for reference.

CHAPTER 7

Female Sleep Specifics: Sleep Disorders, Pain and Mental Health

After learning about the hormone transitions and their relationship with sleep across a woman's lifespan, you would be justified in thinking that women's sleep deserves a break. But no, unfortunately, there are other non-hormonal factors impacting on a woman's sleep over the course of her lifespan and this chapter will highlight some of these issues, starting with sleep disorders.

SLEEP DISORDERS

Updated in 2023, the International Classification of Sleep Disorders (American Academy of Sleep Medicine, 2023) reported six categories of sleep disorder. As mentioned in Chapter 1, these categories are:

- insomnia disorders
- sleep-related breathing disorders
- central disorders of hypersomnolence
- circadian rhythm sleep–wake disorders
- parasomnias
- sleep-related movement disorders.

A detailed description of each disorder is available in the International Classification of Sleep Disorders and (see also American Academy of Sleep Medicine's website signposted at the end of this book), and it is regarded as an essential reference for all clinicians and researchers for accurately diagnosing sleep disorders. Rather than describe every type of sleep disorder, in this chapter I will focus on the primary sleep disorders frequently experienced by women, starting with the common sleep disorder insomnia.

INSOMNIA

Insomnia is particularly prevalent in women as they enter midlife and the menopause transition. Women are twice as likely to suffer from insomnia as men, and predominantly in later life.

As described in Chapter 1, insomnia is a prolonged sleep issue which is distinct from sleep restriction. The basic difference between the two is that with restricted sleep, a person has a *sufficient ability* to fall asleep, but *insufficient opportunity* to do so. Consequently, an individual can fall asleep, but for whatever reason they are not allowing themselves adequate opportunity to get good sleep. Working excessive hours until late into the night is a good example of where a person might experience restricted sleep.

The criteria for insomnia on the other hand include difficulty initiating sleep or maintaining sleep, waking too early (before a desired sleep bout has finished) or non-restorative[1] or poor-quality sleep. Another marker is that the sleep difficulty occurs despite adequate opportunity and circumstances for sleep, and that one or more complaints of daytime impairment are due to the sleep difficulty. A person with insomnia will report significant daytime problems that affect their ability to function at their best, with daytime fatigue, low mood or irritability, and problems with attention or concentration also typically being experienced (Riemann *et al.*, 2023). So, an individual may go to bed at a reasonable time but lack the ability to fall asleep or stay asleep during the night.

Insomniacs, therefore, cannot generate the sleep quantity or quality that they require, despite giving themselves ample time in bed to do so. What's happening to prevent the ability to fall asleep is essentially the brain remaining in a *hyperaroused* state or a position of *readiness* that cannot be 'switched off' and thus inhibits sleep. This is a very different state of mind to normal sleepers, who appear to be able to nod off automatically. Insomnia can be acute or chronic and, in either state,

---

1   Non-restorative sleep is defined as the subjective feeling that sleep has been insufficiently refreshing, often despite the appearance of physiologically normal sleep (Wilkinson & Shapiro, 2013).

significantly affect a person's daytime functioning and overall quality of life. Acute insomnia can exist due to a temporary life or work stress and can be overcome relatively quickly once the stress subsides, but chronic insomnia is a horrible condition to endure and significantly affects quality of life.

Many studies of insomnia relate to a model of *predisposing, precipitating* and *perpetuating factors* (Spielman, 1986). Predisposing factors include childhood trauma or family history. Examples of precipitating factors would be the menopause, mood disorder, medications or psychological stressors. Perpetuating factors tend to relate to inappropriate napping, work, caregiving, parenting, anxiety or irregular sleep schedules. So, for example, a woman with a family history of insomnia (predisposing factor), who is experiencing the menopause transition (precipitating factor) and has an irregular sleep schedule (perpetuating factor) could be a prime candidate for insomnia.

To add to the mix, insomnia has several variants. Numerous definitions exist, but essentially there are three different features of this debilitating sleep disorder. First is difficulty initiating sleep, which is known as *sleep onset insomnia* and can be acute or chronic. Second is difficulty in staying asleep, known as *sleep maintenance insomnia*, which is an inability to stay asleep despite having fallen asleep without a problem. Finally, there is the type of insomnia where an individual just doesn't feel refreshed or restored at all after a night's sleep. Despite being able to fall asleep and stay asleep, they don't feel like they have had a good night's sleep at all, and daytime function is impaired. This is known as *non-restorative sleep*. Unfortunately, a person can experience one or all types of insomnia at any one time. A comprehensive list of insomnia variations, and all sleep disorders, can be found in Thorpy (2012) and more recently in Riemann *et al.* (2023).

The causes of insomnia can be different too. Broadly, there are three categories: it can be *psychological*, a temporary life stress causing some mental stress meaning sleep is affected. Or it could be *pathophysiological*, where a biological reason is causing sleep to be elusive, such as a woman experiencing hot flushes. Or, finally, insomnia could be due to an *environmental* issue – for example, where a person's bedroom is too hot or noisy, or they've had too much to eat or consumed too much caffeine.

Clinicians will typically use the '30, 30, 3 rule' as a guide to determine if an individual is suspected of experiencing insomnia. This means if it takes at least 30 minutes to fall asleep, or *get back* to sleep after waking during the night, and that this is happening at least for three nights a week, for three months or more, then the individual would be a candidate for insomnia interventions. However, three months seems a long time to be enduring poor sleep before seeking help, so if a client is describing persistent sleep issues, I would err on the side of caution and suggest they see a medical practitioner as soon as possible.

Useful strategies to try to combat insomnia fall under clinical intervention, but not always with a need for prescription medicine. A successful non-pharmacological pathway for insomnia can include cognitive behavioural therapy for insomnia (CBT-I). This is widely regarded as the first line of defence in response to the frustrating symptoms of insomnia, ahead of any form of pharmacological intervention, and uses a short, structured and evidence-based approach (Baglioni *et al.*, 2022).

CBT-I is an umbrella term for a few multicomponent treatments to try to help individuals to fall asleep faster, stay asleep and feel more rested during the day (Ellis, personal communication, 2024). Component treatments will include the following: education around sleep hygiene, stimulus control (using the bedroom only to sleep and leaving the bedroom if unable to sleep), sleep restriction (a multistep, multi-week process that initially restricts the amount of time a person spends in bed overnight and then gradually increases that time), relaxation techniques (e.g. meditation), a cognitive element (changing unhelpful thoughts about sleep) and a review where the components are revised to prevent relapse happening (Erten Uyumaz *et al.*, 2021). Table 7.1 highlights the different components of CBT-I treatment.

Table 7.1 The structure of CBT-I components in in-person treatment (adapted from Erten Uyumaz *et al.*, 2021)

Sleep hygiene	Stimulus control	Sleep restriction	Relaxation	Cognitive	Review

Occasionally, CBT-I may not work for an individual. This could be due to it being an unsuitable time for a client to engage with the therapy, or a disconnect between the therapist and the client. Finding a therapist and a form of CBT-I that works for the individual is critical to the success of the intervention, so if clients attempt CBT-I and find it's not helping, suggest that they persevere with another therapist, or mode of CBT-I, until they find good results. Revisiting CBT-I is encouraged before looking into further interventions for insomnia (Gavriloff, 2024), but if an individual really doesn't like CBT-I and is finding it unsuccessful, then they should seek further guidance on insomnia treatment from a medical practitioner, such as, if appropriate, a menopause specialist doctor.

Professor Jason Ellis, an experienced researcher in the field of insomnia, produced a useful resource for acute insomnia, 'Coping with Stress Related Sleep Loss', which may be beneficial for your clients if initial symptoms appear. It focuses on first *detecting* if indeed acute insomnia is present or if it is another sleep disorder or is being caused by something or someone else, then *detaching* from the stressful situation of not falling asleep. For example, the person could find something else to do other than trying to fall asleep until they feel sleepy, such as reading a book or performing some breathing exercises. The final stage is *distracting* from the issue of not falling asleep, as the longer the person lies awake, the harder it is for them to fall asleep. This is where advice such as counting sheep or counting back from 100 has a place. A copy of the leaflet 'Coping with Stress Related Sleep Loss' is available by contacting Professor Jason Ellis (Northumbria University), and is signposted at the end of the book.

There are also some good virtual therapy options for CBT-I available, with different versions offered either as a supplementary tool to face-to-face CBT-I or as standalone treatments. First, there is digital CBT-I, where the digital component is provided as an accompanying tool for in-person treatment to perform post-session assignments. There is also guided digital CBT-I, where the digital medium is provided, such as an app, with a therapist's decision and input on the content and feedback. Finally, there is fully automated digital CBT-I which involves digital programs that use media interactions and are adapted by algorithms (Erten Uyumaz *et al.*, 2021). All have merit and which CBT-I treatment pathway suits a person really comes down to personal preference and what resources are available to them.

The principal advantages of *digital* CBT-I compared to in-person, face-to-face practitioners are the availability of support, bespoke information, innovative avenues for communication and efficient review options for a client's progress (Erten Uyumaz *et al.*, 2021). They aren't without their problems, though, with disadvantages linked to technical issues, a lack of adherence by the client and over-generalization of advice (Erten Uyumaz *et al.*, 2021).

Further, a significant disadvantage with CBT-I, in any form, is access to practitioners. There are very few specialist face-to-face CBT-I practitioners nationwide in the UK, certainly not in every hospital trust, for example. Finding one close to where your client lives may be tricky, and this is where digital therapies may have a place. Equally, there currently is no standardization of credentials for CBT-I delivery, so finding quality-assured practitioners can be difficult. A selection of good training opportunities for CBT-I can be found in the resources section at the end of this book, and a wider description of some sleep education courses is given in Chapter 10.

The good news, as of 2024, is that a digital CBT-I therapy option called Sleepio became available in all NHS trusts in England and Wales. Whilst this is a positive step forward for people to access CBT-I, sadly not everyone has access to the internet. Staggeringly, approximately seven million UK households don't have internet access and four million people in the UK aren't technologically capable to undertake a single basic digital task, for example opening an internet browser (Sleep Charity, 2024). So unfortunately, some demographics may still be at a disadvantage for accessing any form of CBT-I.

In addition to the issue of a lack of CBT-I practitioners, I am fully aware that encouraging a dialogue with clients about their sleep from a medical practitioner's point of view may be opening Pandora's box, as often the correct treatment option isn't available, and the practitioner may not be informed about the potential treatment options.

Limited specialist sleep medics, alongside limited resources or allied practitioners to help those in need of good sleep support, often result in diagnosing a sleep issue where only a limited solution exists, at least in the short term. The most one can do in these situations is use the growing set of education resources and support options, some of which are signposted at the end of this book, and refer appropriately where there is a direct clinical need.

As with most health-related issues, the process to access support can often be slow, but it is better than not doing anything at all.

Similarly, I am aware that suggesting a primary care practitioner or allied health professional has a dialogue about sleep in an already limited consultation time frame, when sleep may not be the principal presenting issue, is challenging. However, in order to create change and ultimately improve public health, I believe encouraging such a dialogue is better than doing nothing.

OTHER SLEEP DISORDERS

As mentioned in Chapter 1, women may suffer other sleep disorders such as restless leg syndrome (RLS), periodic limb movement (PLM) and a form of sleep-disordered breathing, sleep apnoea. Both RLS and PLM are relatively rare and can often be experienced alongside other sleep disorders, such as insomnia (Riemann *et al.*, 2023).

Restless leg syndrome and periodic limb movement

Restless leg syndrome occurs when uncomfortable sensations in the legs, such as itching, prickling, pulling or crawling, create an overwhelming urge to move the legs. Periodic limb movement involves repetitive jerking, cramping or twitching of their lower limbs during sleep, usually occurring every five to 90 seconds for up to an hour (Bryan & Peters, 2024; Pacheco and Wells, 2024). Treatment requires clinical intervention, so advise clients to get some guidance from a medical practitioner. Also be aware that sometimes these conditions don't fall under sleep disorders and are often described as musculoskeletal conditions, so it can sometimes be hard to find the correct treatment option.

Sleep-disordered breathing

Sleep-disordered breathing (SDB) is a common sleep disorder. As described in Chapter 1, this is a broad spectrum of sleep-related breathing disorders, including obstructive sleep apnoea (OSA), central sleep apnoea, as well as sleep-related hypoventilation (too slow or shallow breathing) and hypoxemia (low levels of oxygen in the blood).

The most prevalent sleep-disordered breathing issue is obstructive sleep apnoea, with estimates of 12 to 20 per cent of the world's population being affected. Those who smoke, are overweight or lead a sedentary lifestyle are at a higher risk for sleep-disordered breathing.

With OSA, the airway partially or fully collapses during sleep, result-ing in disrupted breathing and a lack of oxygen. Central sleep apnoea (CSA) on the other hand is caused by a momentary lack of communi-cation between brain and breathing muscles, leading to an increased number of reductions or pauses in breathing during sleep.

Sleep apnoea causes breathing to slow or stop for seconds, or even minutes at a time, and significantly affects sleep quality, resulting in excessive daytime sleepiness. Figure 7.1 describes the cycle of sleep apnoea, which can occur from ten to up to 300 times a night, hence why an individual will suffer a restless night's sleep and experience extreme daytime sleepiness the following day.

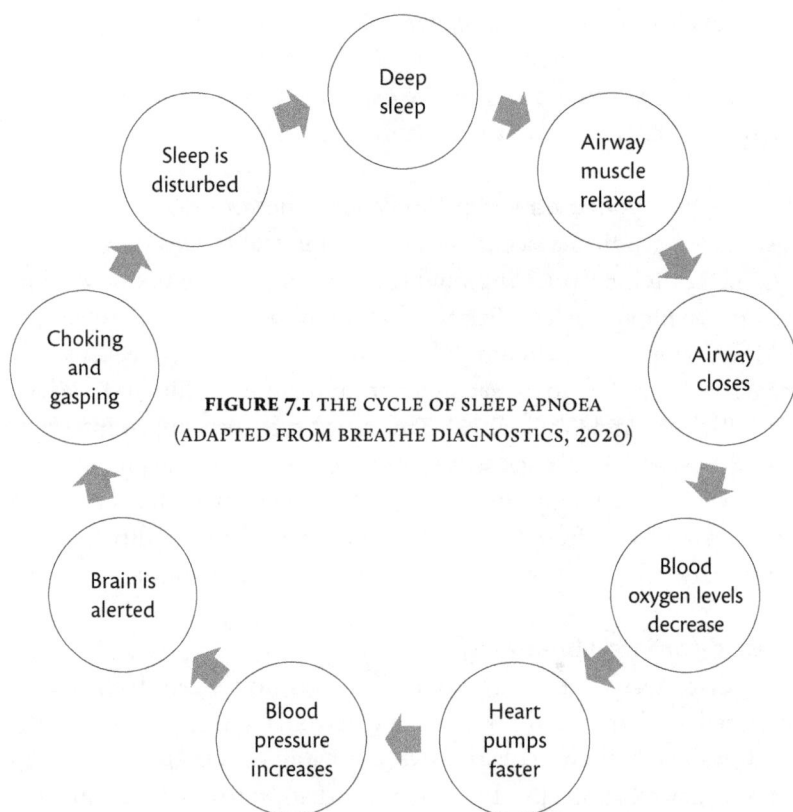

FIGURE 7.1 THE CYCLE OF SLEEP APNOEA (ADAPTED FROM BREATHE DIAGNOSTICS, 2020)

Obstructive sleep apnoea is characterized by a restricted airway due to an increased body mass, causing an enlarged neck circumference, put-ting subsequent pressure on the airway. It is more common in men, but can increase its manifestation in women – often, but not only, pregnant women or those undergoing the menopause transition. Progesterone possibly has a protective effect on respiration and, as we have seen, declines in the menopause transition phase. Muscle tone is also lost due to the decline in hormones during the menopause transition, and therefore a woman's airway can sometimes collapse (Franklin *et al.*, 2013; Wimms *et al.*, 2016; Haufe & Leeners, 2023).

The restricted airway in OSA causes temporary pauses in breathing during sleep, resulting in symptoms such as loud snoring, making choking sounds or having difficulty with breathing during sleep, any or all of which are likely to waken the sleeper. More atypical yet common sleep apnoea symptoms in women are insomnia, restless leg syndrome, a dry mouth, depression, excessive daytime sleepiness, headaches (particularly morning headaches) and muscle pain (Valipour *et al.*, 2007; Wimms *et al.*, 2016).

Both obstructive and central sleep apnoea require clinical intervention and require referral to a specialist clinician. If you suspect sleep-disordered breathing and are referring your client for specialist support, it is often useful to ask the individual to complete a couple of clinically recognized questionnaires to help inform decision making around the diagnosis. The Epworth Sleepiness Scale (Johns, 1990), described in Chapter 2, would be useful here, as would the STOPBang questionnaire used by respiratory medicine practitioners in the assessment of sleep-disordered breathing, and both can be found on the British Snoring and Sleep Apnoea Association's website among other places (both questionnaires are signposted at the end of this book).

Treatment for obstructive sleep apnoea usually involves making lifestyle changes, such as losing weight and stopping smoking. An intervention involving a device known as a continuous positive airway pressure (CPAP) machine is also recommended as a treatment option for adults with moderate or severe symptomatic obstructive sleep apnoea (NICE, 2021). The NHS offers information on this form of treatment and is signposted at the end of this book.

It is estimated that 1.5 million people in the UK suffer from sleep apnoea, yet only 330,000 are being treated, which illustrates the scale of the problem and, more worryingly, the number of people who are regularly functioning on significantly restricted sleep. This has implications not only for their health but for the safety of wider society and industry if they are employed in roles where excessive daytime sleepiness could be dangerous (see Chapter 10 for discussion around safety-critical industries and sleep).

The British Sleep Society and the Royal Society of Medicine offer lots of information and training in relation to dentistry and respiratory medicine to help patients with sleep-disordered breathing. More information can be found on their websites, and these are signposted at the end of this book. Additionally, Hope2Sleep is a charity focused on raising awareness of sleep apnoea and has lots of useful information about the condition on their website (also signposted at the end of this book).

Specific expertise is required for the diagnosis and treatment of sleep disorders. As women can potentially suffer from sleep disorders throughout their life, it is pertinent to have an awareness of what the disorders might be, possible interventions and a knowledge of where to signpost if necessary. This chapter has aimed to provide an overview of the leading sleep disorders that women may experience throughout their lifetime. What follows in the remainder of this chapter are some circumstances where a woman's sleep may also be restricted, although not necessarily during a hormone transition phase or because of a specific sleep disorder, that can be equally challenging to a woman's ability to get good sleep.

PAIN AND FEMALE SLEEP

Pain is universal to both males and females. There is plenty of evidence to suggest that sleep and pain are related, but the exact mechanisms around the relationship remain unknown, other than the fact that the relationship is, like many other factors related to sleep, reciprocal, intricate and multifaceted (Finan, Goodin & Smith, 2013; Haack *et al.*, 2020).

In terms of chronic pain (pain lasting from three to six months or more) and sleep, chronic pain has an established impact on sleep. Sleep disturbances occur simultaneously with chronic pain and exacerbate pain symptoms, with up to 88 per cent of chronic pain patients reporting coexisting sleep problems (Rouhi *et al.*, 2023). These sleep issues are typically characterized by reduced sleep duration, fragmented sleep, increased awakenings and decreased sleep efficiency. Studies allude to the fact that sleep restriction can cause *hyperalgesic* changes (Haack *et al.*, 2020). This is where the individual has an abnormally heightened sensitivity to pain.

However, determining the exact cause in relation to poor sleep, such as a loss of sleep architecture or total sleep time, is difficult.

Women can be predisposed to experience poorer sleep in relation to pain at various points throughout their lives – for example, menstruation or postpartum pain. Certainly, women have increased pain sensitivity and are more vulnerable to chronic pain conditions, such as migraine, heartburn and arthritis (Pacheco & Rehman, 2023), all of which can have a concomitant effect on sleep health.

There is also evidence to suggest women experience pain differently to men after the onset of puberty (Vincent and Tracey, 2008). The reason? Hormones (again). Compared to males, whose sex hormone, testosterone, has an analgesic (pain-relieving) effect, woman are, generally, more likely to experience pain than men, and this again primarily can be related to the ovarian hormones oestrogen and progesterone. Whilst social and psychological factors certainly play a role in the differences of the prevalence and incidence of pain, biological differences, such as hormones, probably underlie these effects. For example, the cyclical nature of the ovarian hormones throughout the menstrual cycle (described in Chapter 4) has been related to a different clinical response in how women experience and tolerate pain, and its intensity, over the course of a menstrual cycle. Similarly, women with endometriosis suffer a lower pain threshold if they have also had poor sleep (Nunes, Ferreira & Bahamondes, 2015). This isn't to say men don't experience a heightened pain response due to a lack of sleep, more that women are predisposed to experience pain due to the interaction of their ovarian hormones and pain.

Despite evidence for female ovarian hormones affecting pain, the relationship is far from straightforward (Vincent & Tracey, 2008; Haack *et al.*, 2020). The collective effect of these hormones on pain is complex and likely depends on the interaction between the hormones and the extent of their fluctuation, rather than absolute hormone levels.

As with any hormone interaction in the human body, many factors need to be considered, not least the type of relationship with pain. For example, is it dose dependent – are woman more susceptible to pain with higher or lower levels of the particular ovarian hormone? Does the hormone have an interplay outside of its primary role in the reproductive system? We know ovarian hormones do play a part in other areas of the body, so it seems feasible that they will interact with a woman's pain experience throughout her biological system – for example, nervous system and immune function.

What is clear is that all three factors interlink: pain, sleep and female hormones. Sleep plays a part in the ability to tolerate pain, particularly in women, and women are more likely to experience pain throughout their life. Tie the two together and it is unsurprising that female sleep and pain have a strong reciprocal relationship.

Despite consistent data showing that sleep and pain are related, there is a problem with limited longitudinal studies investigating sleep disturbances as a possible clinical cause of chronic pain. Because of the effect of pain and sleep problems on quality of life, investigating how sleep and pain are connected is fundamental to improving health outcomes through better treatments and prevention strategies (Andersen *et al.*, 2018; Haack *et al.*, 2020). However, in women, the likelihood of coexisting health conditions, and fluctuating hormones, particularly during the menopause, makes is difficult to study sleep. Therefore, much more research is needed to improve both the understanding of the complex area of women's sleep and pain and the subsequent management of painful conditions (Vincent & Tracey, 2008).

The challenging symptoms of being in regular pain may also have an impact on a woman's mental health. For example, if a woman in pain experiences even more discomfort, then they are more likely to feel depressed or anxious about it and then enter a vicious cycle of poor sleep, pain and emotional disturbance. This is another area of women's sleep to consider since it interacts with many of the areas we have already discussed – for example, adolescence, postpartum or the menopause transition. Given the propensity of women to experience certain mental health disorders, whether due to life stressors or phase of life or both, it's important to consider mental health and sleep in the lifespan of a woman.

MENTAL HEALTH AND SLEEP

Before we get into the detail of mental health and sleep, I feel it's important to reiterate I am not a psychologist, and I am highly aware of where my professional boundaries lie in this area. However, when advising and educating about sleep health, there is no escaping a conversation around mental health and sleep. The two are inextricably linked. Principally, I will provide the headlines around the reciprocal relationship between the two. Where clients need a mental health intervention, or at least a referral, I signpost to several different avenues of support, such as the client's GP, a clinical psychologist or CBT-I specialist, alongside various virtual resources signposted at the end of this book. I also provide information about practical interventions which may help *in addition* to a more clinical pathway of support. No practical solution will 'fix' a sleep disorder or clinical mental health condition. Both require clinical expertise and intervention.

At this point it's also important to recognize the difference between poor mental health and a mental health condition. Both have a reciprocal relationship with sleep, but the extent of the multidisciplinary support required for each issue can be quite different. As described in Chapter 5, poor mental health is a state that has a negative impact on the way a person thinks, feels or behaves, whereas mental ill health is the degree and length of time the difficulties experienced impact a person's wellbeing and functioning and when the impact of the person's poor mental health is to the extent that it could be a diagnosable mental health condition (Mental Health First Aid England first aid course, 2023, personal communication).

Mental health and sleep have a reciprocal relationship in much the same way as other aspects of health and wellbeing and sleep do. Many people with a mental health condition report poor sleep and there are a whole host of mental health conditions linked to sleep – for example, anxiety disorders, depression, paranoia and psychosis (Robotham, 2011). Most people experiencing poor mental health to some degree will experience poor sleep as well, or vice versa. From the Great British Sleep Survey (*The Guardian*, 2011), it was reported that four out of five long-term poor sleepers experience low mood and are seven times more likely to feel helpless and five times more likely to feel alone.

Studies of mental health and sleep are many and varied. A recent comprehensive review by Scott and colleagues (2021) would be a good place to start if you are particularly interested in delving into this area in more detail. In terms of women and mental health, longitudinal studies have demonstrated an association between the menopause transition and an increase in depressive symptoms (Vivian-Taylor & Hickey, 2014). Unsurprisingly, during the teenage years, sleep disturbances are regarded as high-risk factors for adolescent mental health problems, such as depression and anxiety (Qiu & Morales-Muñoz, 2022). Similarly, restricted sleep with a newborn baby is a non-negotiable, which therefore, unfortunately, can sometimes lead to postpartum mental health issues for both parents.

Perinatal mental ill health encompasses mental health conditions that can affect parents during pregnancy or within the first postnatal year. These conditions include antenatal and postpartum depression and anxiety, postpartum psychosis, obsessive compulsive disorder (OCD), tokophobia (an extreme fear of pregnancy and childbirth), birth trauma or post-traumatic stress disorder (PTSD) (PANDAS Foundation UK, 2024). Certainly, postpartum depression is related to sleep loss, as described in Chapter 5. Sleep loss during the postpartum phase can result in a woman feeling exhausted, impatient, having a lower ability to concentrate and an overall lower quality of life, all of which can contribute to an increased risk for postpartum depression (Lewis *et al.*, 2018). Signposting for organizations that can help if you feel a client is living with a form of postpartum mental ill health is available at the end of this book.

The catalogue of mental health disorders and associated poor sleep health that women may suffer throughout their lifespan increases the need for more awareness and additional support for women during challenging times in their life when their sleep is compromised. It also highlights the point that many mental health conditions don't arise in isolation. There may be comorbidities that may influence one another, in addition to the state of an individual's sleep. For example, if a woman is experiencing depression and/or anxiety, then their sleep will certainly suffer. The lack of sleep then also influences other important aspects of wellbeing, such as perception of pain, which, as I have previously discussed, may also be a risk for sleep disturbance. This can be particularly problematic for women experiencing some of the sleep-restricting symptoms of, for example, menses or endometriosis. Similarly, if a woman is affected by obesity and associated sleep-disordered breathing, they may also go on to experience a mental health condition such as depression or anxiety. Stress, another significant factor in mental health and sleep, also has a reciprocal relationship with sleep, and we saw in Chapter 2 how stress and sleep are related through the body's physiological response to stress.

In March 2020, the Mental Health Foundation commissioned two surveys on sleep and mental health from YouGov: one of 4437 UK adults aged 18 and over and another of 2412 British teenagers aged between 13 and 19. They reported that nearly half (48%) of adults and two-thirds of teenagers (66%) agreed that sleeping badly had a negative effect on their mental health. The Mental Health Foundation also reported that characteristics of a workplace affect sleep and mental health. They found that 37 per cent of working adults stated that their occupation (e.g. workload, problems with colleagues and worries about job security) reduced the amount of control they felt they had over their sleep. Employers should ensure they support good sleep and good mental health at work by promoting, for example, a choice of shift and a good work–life balance, offering healthy sleep programmes to staff and consulting experts and worker representatives to develop flexible work schedules. This is where some of my sleep health education webinars are particularly impactful as they offer employers and employees an opportunity to better understand sleep and therefore make changes, not only to be more productive in the workplace but also perhaps improve their overall physical and mental wellbeing.

The good news is there are plenty of strategies to help manage not only mental health conditions but also the associated sleep issues. As ever with sleep, these issues can be complex and individualized, and may require medical intervention. Traditionally, poor sleep wasn't always seen as a contributory causal factor in mental health problems. The situation was more that poor sleep was viewed as a symptom, or consequence, of mental health disorders, and consequently allocated a lower priority in the treatment pathway of patients with such disorders. However, whilst the causal relationship between sleep and mental health is difficult to decipher, the link between the two cannot be ignored. Further research has since reported that given the fact that interventions to help improve sleep can have a positive effect on mental health problems, the link is more likely causal (Scott *et al.*, 2021). There could also potentially be a dose–response relationship where greater improvements in sleep quality could lead to greater improvements in mental health (Scott *et al.*, 2021).

Future practice supporting those with mental health conditions will, it is hoped, take a more holistic view towards the management of such illnesses and include interventions to improve sleep as part of the treatment pathway. Not least, the treatment of disrupted sleep should be given a higher priority in mental health provision (Freeman *et al.*, 2017).

COST-OF-LIVING CRISIS AND SLEEP

You can't really write a book about sleep and not mention the current cost-of-living crisis, particularly in relation to the relationship between sleep and mental health. The Money and Mental Health Policy Institute (2022) reported that the cost-of-living squeeze could cause a national mental health crisis, with a staggering 11 million UK adults saying they feel 'unable to cope' due to rising costs. They also found that 59 per cent of UK adults reported that the cost-of-living crisis had had a negative impact on their mental health, such as feeling anxious, depressed or hopeless.

According to the British Association for Counselling and Psychotherapy (BACP), concerns over the cost-of-living crisis are causing a decline in people's mental health, with 52 per cent of therapists reporting a rise in clients' insomnia over money worries (Psychreg, 2024). The Money and Mental Health Policy Institute (2022) advise three ways to help cope with the stress of the cost-of-living crisis: (1) stay in touch with friends and family; (2) get help to support your financial situation; and (3) do things to help mental health – for example, get good sleep and exercise.

BED POVERTY

In line with the cost-of-living crisis, there is a huge problem worldwide with bed poverty, including in the UK, with 30 per cent of families without adequate beds. Bed, or more generally sleep, poverty affects people who can't afford decent bedding (or housing) and those working long hours, continental shifts and multiple occupations (Mycroft, 2022). Bed poverty encompasses anything from broken beds and damaged bedding, having to share a bed or room or even sleeping on the floor, to not having sufficient bedding or not being able to afford to wash bedding (Cooper & Mullen, 2023).

I realize, in advising on sleep health and educating people about it, that it is not always easy for people to access the right sleep system for them or their family. When I talk to people about improving their sleep, usually to help performance, be it in sport or work, the issue of bed poverty isn't really considered. Yet for far too many people in the UK, it is an issue, and it has a significant effect on their overall health.

According to the UK children's charity Barnardo's, most of the families they support have been affected by the cost-of-living crisis. With very little, if any, disposable income, families struggle to provide the basic essential items, such as gas, electricity or food, and so furniture simply isn't a priority purchase. Some organizations are trying to reach out with some great initiatives to help those in need. More information can be found on the website of Zarach, a charity committed to helping children and families who are living in poverty crisis, or Barnardo's and the Sleep Charity websites (see the resources section at the end of the book).

Whilst the cost-of-living crisis and bed poverty are wider issues than just sleep across a woman's' lifespan, without a doubt both will impact significantly on a woman's sleep if she is experiencing difficulties in either area, or both.

SLEEP AND THE COVID-19 PANDEMIC

Another factor related to mental health and sleep has been the recent Covid-19 pandemic (2020–2021) and its subsequent effect on sleep, both long term and during the pandemic itself. It would be remiss of me to write a book about sleep and not consider the impact the pandemic has had on the world's sleep patterns, particularly when we observe the impact of the pandemic on women's sleep.

Clearly, the pandemic caused international distress on a grand scale, with countries adopting different policies involving city lockdowns, border control, online teaching and social distancing to slow down the Covid-19 infection rate (Alimoradi *et al.*, 2022).

Mental health suffered greatly during and following the Covid-19 pandemic, with associated sleep health being significantly affected. In 2021, BBC Worklife reported the disastrous consequences for sleep brought about by the pandemic and its ongoing effect on people's lives. For instance, they reported that the word 'insomnia' was googled more in 2020 than it had ever been before. The phenomenon 'coronasomnia', the experience of insomnia linked to the stress of life during Covid-19, suggests how impactful the virus was on our sleep (Lufkin, 2021). Unfortunately, at the time of writing, this is an ongoing issue.

A study from the University of Southampton showed that in the UK in 2020, the number of people experiencing insomnia rose from one in six to one in four, with more sleep problems in communities including, notably, mothers, along with essential workers and ethnically diverse communities. In China, insomnia rates rose from nearly 15 per cent to 20 per cent during peak lockdown (Morin & Carrier, 2021), and a disturbing prevalence of insomnia was also observed in countries such as Italy (Bacaro *et al.*, 2020) and Greece (Voitsidis *et al.*, 2020; Falkingham, Evandrou & Vlachantoni, 2022).

Since Covid-19, one in three UK residents have been sleeping less than before, whilst one in five have been sleeping more than usual. Much of the emerging research suggests experiences during the Covid-19 pandemic in the UK were very different for men and women. Given that women are more likely to suffer insomnia, report psychological distress and work in a healthcare profession, a relatively high prevalence of sleep problems emerged during the Covid-19 pandemic that imposed a disproportionate impact on women compared to men (Falkingham *et al.*, 2022).

As women make up a large proportion of frontline workers in education, social and health care, their experiences of sleep during the pandemic were different to those of men and they were potentially more vulnerable. The proportion of women in general losing sleep over worry before the Covid-19 pandemic was 18.9 per cent, rising to 31 per cent during the pandemic. By comparison, the number of men reporting sleep loss increased from 11.9 per cent to 16.5 per cent during the Covid-19 lockdown (Falkingham *et al.*, 2022).

Added to the mix were women with young children whose sleep loss alarmingly doubled during the first few weeks of the Covid-19 pandemic. Of women with children aged zero to four years, 19.5 per cent experienced sleep loss over worry before the pandemic, compared to a staggering 40 per cent during the first four weeks of the lockdown. For women with school children aged five to eighteen, sleep loss also rose, from 21.7 per cent to 38 per cent (Falkingham *et al.*, 2022). This isn't to say men didn't experience sleep issues during the Covid-19 pandemic, but for women the impact on sleep appears to have been quite dramatic.

Technology didn't help either, with the immediate availability of news reports, thanks to the internet, access to devices in the home and rolling news items. How news channels continuously and routinely reported on daily deaths and on the number of cumulative infected cases of Covid-19, both in the UK and globally, undoubtedly generated the anxiety and stress that led to sleep disturbances during the pandemic.

During this time, there was also an increase in people's disturbed sleep due to their amplified behaviour around social media use. Consequently, the pandemic enhanced the mental health issues surrounding sleep as people's lives underwent immeasurable change. A reduction in social channels, a concomitant increase in family responsibilities and work pressures, and an overall lack of routine all contributed to sleep-related problems throughout the pandemic.

There was also the impact on sleep of contracting the virus itself, with post-Covid-19 infection sleep issues, such as insomnia, still being observed in the present day. Alarmingly, although perhaps unsurprisingly, among the 200 different symptoms reported after Covid-19 infection, insomnia is one of the most common (Hoang *et al.*, 2024).

Benefits to certain industries, such as pharmaceutical and technological, as a result of sleep issues during and after the pandemic have been great. The pandemic acted as a catalyst of significant life stress, impacting on sleep issues on a global scale, and therefore resulted in intense market growth for companies invested in sleep disorders such as insomnia. Pharmaceutical and technology industries make billions of dollars by taking advantage of the rise in sleep disorders. According to market research firm Imarc, the global insomnia market will make $5.1 billion in 2022 and increase to $6.1 billion by 2028. That includes spending on prescription drugs, over-the-counter sleep aids, medical devices and various types of therapy (Levy, 2022).

The adverse impacts of long-term lockdown on mental health were harsh for all populations, not least for women, and further work needs to be done regarding the fallout on sleep quality and quantity after the Covid-19 pandemic.

If you have a client who expresses concerns over a mental health condition, or you are worried for them, do try to refer them to their GP for further support. If you are not medically trained, or don't work in the domain of mental health, but wish to develop your knowledge further, there are some very good resources and courses through Mental Health First Aid England which are signposted at the end of this book.

CHAPTER 8

Female Sleep Specifics: Shift Work and Carer Responsibilities

As described previously, there are a host of other areas outside of the typical hormone transitions where a woman's sleep may be challenged throughout her lifespan. This chapter will focus on aspects relating to shift work and other responsibilities or conditions a woman may experience throughout her life that may impact her sleep.

SHIFT WORK AND FEMALE SLEEP

Nearly 12 per cent of the British workforce perform night shifts, with approximately one in five employees working some form of non-traditional shift (working outside regular daytime hours) throughout the industrialized world (Wickwire *et al.*, 2017).

Shift work is common in many safety-critical sectors including transportation and healthcare (Houses of Parliament, 2018). It can encompass many different types of working model, all of which will compromise nighttime sleep. To what extent depends on how well shift patterns are managed and the proactivity of the shift worker to utilize coping strategies around the night work.

Whilst the shift work population is predominantly male, a growing sector in shift work is health and social care, of which women comprise much of the workforce (77%). In fact, 21 per cent of all occupations held by women are in this sector (Francis-Devine & Hutton, 2024).

According to the Trades Union Congress (2018), the number of people working night shifts in in the UK in 2018 reached more than three million, a 5 per cent increase since 2013, with women accounting for two-thirds (66.8%) of the increase. Therefore, for a large proportion of women, night shift work can be a significant contributing factor to the quality of their sleep.

Working night shifts involves physical and mental fatigue. Physical fatigue is exacerbated by increased work duration and readily reduced by rest breaks. Mental fatigue is also impaired with increased work duration and reduced by rest breaks, but it doesn't just accumulate and dissipate progressively with time on and off work. Other factors, especially time of day and the durations of wakefulness and prior sleep, also have a significant effect on mental fatigue (Gurubhagavatula *et al.*, 2021). Therefore, mental fatigue is associated with considerable risks to shift work employees, employers, and wider society.

Shift work is linked with an increased risk of sleep problems, occupational and driving accidents, and long-term health conditions (Houses of Parliament, 2018). Acute risks of shift work include reductions in performance, effectiveness and productivity and increased errors, to name a few. More long-term risks include degraded physical and mental health and reduced individual and community wellbeing, not to mention the economic losses (Gurubhagavatula *et al.*, 2021) (more on sleep and the economy in Chapter 10).

Shift work is well known to affect a person's sleep patterns and sleep health. The primary issue with shift work and sleep is the disruption to the body's natural rhythm. I described in Chapter 2 how humans have their own internal (circadian) rhythm for many physiological states, and the sleep-and-wake state is a principal one. Working night shifts upsets the body's sleep–wake circadian rhythm to the point that the body is in opposition with itself. That is, a person is awake when naturally they should be asleep and asleep when they should naturally be awake. Shift workers must fight the body's biological rhythms to try to stay awake at night to work but then may feel sleepy in the day when the body 'expects' to be alert.

Typical issues relating to shift work and sleep are fatigue, managing sleep needs, work patterns around family life and maintaining a healthy lifestyle, including good eating habits. These are not exclusive to women working shifts, but a significant challenge to those who are (Harrington, 2001).

In rare cases, a more severe response to shift work can manifest, known as shift work sleep disorder (SWSD). This typically occurs when an individual has a history of chronic shift work. It is different from the regular physical or mental fatigue experienced from working shifts, in that the symptoms are excessive and falling asleep is an issue no matter when the individual is working or what time of day it is. It is a circadian rhythm disorder that affects people who work non-traditional hours, such as different shifts, or work at night, and is due to either changes in the circadian system or a misalignment between a person's circadian rhythm and the external or environmental factors that affect the timing or duration of sleep – for example, light exposure or mealtimes. Symptoms involve a persistent or recurrent sleep disturbance occurring when a shift worker has difficulty adjusting to different sleep–wake schedules, has sleep disturbances before or after their shift, and/or excessive sleepiness and fatigue during their shifts. An individual may also experience microsleeps (periods of sleep that last from a few to several seconds), mental health issues such as depression, a lack of energy and difficulty concentrating (Wickwire *et al.*, 2017).

Many shift workers often feel like they haven't had enough sleep and, though they may sleep well, often find themselves lethargic and irritable and have difficulty concentrating. For people with shift work sleep disorder, this becomes a continuing problem and begins to interfere with family and social functioning and occupational performance, causing distress or harm. Potentially, this could increase the risk of a myriad of issues, such as chronic sleep disturbance, cognitive impairment and depression.

In addition to the adverse health consequences and diminished quality of life at the individual level, shift work disorder incurs significant costs to employers through reduced workplace performance and increased work-related errors and accidents (Wickwire *et al.*, 2017).

Treatment for shift work sleep disorder is difficult since the individual usually can't change their mode of employment. The condition requires clinical input, alongside lifestyle changes, such as maintaining regular routines when off shift and avoiding caffeine intake, to help manage some of the symptoms. An individual should seek medical advice if they feel they may be experiencing this disorder.

Women working shifts and carrying a potentially greater share of domestic and family responsibilities, alongside possible age-related sleep issues such as sleep-disordered breathing, means that women's sleep health and shift work can have a negative relationship. Women undertaking shift work are more likely to suffer certain diseases, including certain cancers, such as breast cancer. Further, there does seem to be some evidence of an adverse reproductive effect (Chung, Wolf & Shapiro, 2009). Menstrual disruption (cycles less than 25 days or greater than 31 days), infertility (time-to-pregnancy exceeding 12 months) and early spontaneous pregnancy loss (less than 25 weeks) have been associated with shift work (Stocker *et al.*, 2014), though the evidence for this is conflicting and sparse, and the results are ambiguous (Harrington, 2001; Bonde, 2012). Nevertheless, it seems prudent to accept that shift work carries a relative risk to women trying to conceive or who are pregnant, and therefore should be managed accordingly.

Despite the risks to a person's sleep and overall health, demand for shift work is not going to fade given the industrialization of modern society and society's need for services and emergency cover, the technical necessity for maintaining continuous process industries such as pharmaceutical or food production, and the economic need for preventing factories, manufacturing or production plants from becoming unproductive (Harrington, 2001).

The key to helping people manage shift work lies in coping strategies. By this I mean employers designing workplace environments and shift scheduling schemes that lead to the least disruption to mental, physical and social wellbeing (Harrington, 2001). The American Academy of Sleep Medicine and the Sleep Research Society (Gurubhagavatula *et al.*, 2021) published some guiding principles for determining work shift duration and addressing the effects of work shift duration on performance. This is a useful document if you are looking for more information around shift work and its management. It essentially breaks down the management of shift work into multiple factors. To name a few: inadequate sleep (e.g. restricted sleep opportunity) and internal factors (e.g. the circadian rhythm and biological traits), along with external or occupation demands (e.g. family life or workload and stress). These factors (and others) contribute to the guiding principles of decision making to mitigate any health and safety risks of the employees working the shifts (Gurubhagavatula *et al.*, 2021). Fundamentally, sleep strategies form part of the guiding principles through internal and external factors.

Interventions to negate the effects of working shifts are various and include optimizing shift schedules, facilitating rest breaks, screening for sleep disorders and raising awareness around managing shift work and sleep in employers and employees (Houses of Parliament, 2018). It is no surprise that Health and Safety law contains many specific requirements covering shift work. The Working Time Regulations Act 1998 made it the law that employees and workers have the right to rest during the working day through rest breaks, working week (rest between working days) and the year (holiday entitlement). Shift worker breaks may be devised slightly differently to normal office hours, but the fact remains it is illegal for employers not to provide a rest break when an employee is working on shift.

There are some practical strategies an individual can utilize to help prioritize and protect their sleep health when working shift patterns. It is important that a person accepts the fact that sleep is individualized: we all have different sleep needs and sleep associations. Shift work can be hard and there is no 'quick fix', but incorporating it into daily life in accordance with other aspects is one way to manage the daily circadian rhythm disruption. Table 8.1 highlights some tips that may help clients who work shifts, but also advise them to seek medical support if they are concerned about their sleep around their shift patterns.

Table 8.1 Top tips for shift work and sleep

Shift work top tips*	
Breaks	Regular breaks are important
	Where possible, take breaks in a different environment
	Provision of rest rooms can help
	Access to healthy food
	Sleep education/support
Post shift	Driving can be risky
	Use public transport or a taxi if possible
	If appropriate, it can be useful to do some light physical activity briefly before a journey
	Delay journey if feeling sleepy
	Pull over safely if feeling sleepy
	In daylight, wear sunglasses if possible

Sleep extension (napping)	Needs a thorough risk assessment
	Appropriate facilities are required
	After final night shift, aim for a short morning nap and try to keep to 'normal' sleep and mealtimes
	Use appropriately, e.g. do not use in environments where important decisions, particularly safety-critical ones, could be impaired by sleepiness
Bedroom environment	Make it conducive to sleep
	Make sure bed is comfortable, including pillows and bedding
	Try to follow a wind-down routine
	Keep temperature cool: approximately 18–20°C
	Keep lighting low
	Avoid watching TV/screen activity beyond sleep time
	Blackout curtains/blinds/eye masks/ear plugs may help
	Consider using white noise to mask out background noise
	Relaxation activities, e.g. take a bath
	Put a do-not-disturb sign on the door
	Leave mobile phones in the living space
	Ask bed partner to not wake you when they get up. Can they get dressed in another room? Or if there is a spare room, can that be used for shift worker sleep?
	Bedtime routine from environmental cues, e.g. darken the bedroom, rather than take cues from what time it is
Nutrition	Plan meals around the shift
	Choose foods that are easy to digest
	Avoid sugary foods
	Drink plenty of water
	Avoid excessive caffeine overnight
	No alcohol (before or on shift)
	Minimize eating large meals between midnight and 6 a.m. and opt for healthy snacks
	Have something light to eat; don't go to bed hungry
Routine	Exposure to bright light when waking
	Good lifestyle can negate some of the impact of shift work
	Resume usual daily patterns; physical activity is important
	Aim to stick to a regular routine with each shift, go to bed at the same time and wake at the same time – consistency is important
	Avoid spending long periods of time awake in bed
	Have short lie-ins and go to bed slightly earlier first night post shift

Note: Some of these are generic top tips for good sleep and not solely linked to shift work

It should be noted that the consequences for a woman's sleep health from working shifts are often not in isolation. Additional factors such as family and home responsibilities, as well as the aforementioned hormone transition phases and age-related sleep disorders, can mean the sleep health of women who work shifts is significantly compromised and not solely due to the fact that their occupation involves shift work. Women are also more likely to experience restricted sleep due to caregiving responsibilities.

CARER RESPONSIBILITIES

In the UK, the average age of having children is increasing. In 2021, the average age of mothers was 30.9 years, not old by any means, but this figure has been steadily rising in recent decades (Office for National Statistics, 2021). Often women find themselves in the 'sandwich generation' of caring for a young family whilst also having the responsibility of older parents needing support. Combine this with the responsibilities of working and it is easy to see how a woman's sleep may be hampered.

Caring is, of course, also work – even if unpaid. This can include caring for children or elderly relatives and all the emotional labour of running a home: remembering everything from birthday parties to dustbin day, packing lunches and sport kits and ensuring domestic supplies never run short! Ironically, a woman may find herself in this position whilst in the phase of her life when perimenopause symptoms may be appearing. A marvellous double, or even triple, whammy for potential sleep issues!

Much more research is required to fully interpret the impact of life-cycle events on a woman's sleep parameters. Studies to date observing sleep across the lifespan of women have tended to use both subjective (survey) and objective (polysomnography) techniques, but have tended to be of small sample size with diverse methodologies. Without a doubt, a better understanding of the evolution of sleep across a woman's lifespan may lead to more effective therapies that positively impact on women's health and quality of life. The following chapters will provide some insight into some of the practical strategies for obtaining good sleep health and suggest future directions for sleep practice for women and wider society.

CHAPTER 9

Strategies for Good Sleep Health

The recent popularity and interest in sleep means that 'a good night's sleep' is now, more than ever, on people's radar. Given the global societal problem of poor sleep, never before has there been such a need for people to take proactive consideration of their own sleep practices.

Sleep strategies are multicomponent in that there is a myriad of practical approaches an individual can trial to aid sleep. This chapter will cover the principal elements of a good sleep strategy, from establishing a good sleep routine to sleep extension, sleep systems and the sleep environment, nutrition and physical activity, and some contemporary sleep aids.

The essence of achieving good sleep health is having the *ability to generate* good sleep and the *opportunity* to sleep. That is, a person should ideally create an environment where sleep pressure is high (evening) and body time cues are strong and aligned to the body's circadian rhythms of sleep and wake (light/dark cycle); they should also ensure that any pre-sleep arousal is detected and detracted and distracted from (J. Ellis, personal communication, 2024) (remember in Chapter 2, I discussed sleep regulation through two principal mechanisms – sleep pressure and the relationship of the human body's circadian rhythm with the light/dark cycle). In short, sleep health is about ensuring there is a focus on prioritizing, personalizing, valuing and protecting the sleep window (Espie, 2022a), to provide an individual with ample opportunity to gain their personal daily required amount of sleep.

As I mentioned in Chapter 2, it's unrealistic to be idealistic about sleep: the perfect sleep opportunity doesn't present itself on a nightly basis. Instead, try to advise clients to aim for their optimal sleep quality and quantity as much as possible. Being pragmatic and accepting that sleep isn't always going to be 'perfect' is a better approach than being ignorant of the many benefits of good sleep practices.

A question I frequently ask my clients who don't have a sleep disorder but who do struggle with poor sleep is 'Have you ever considered what your strategy is to get to sleep? Have you indeed got one?' Typically, the answer is 'no'. Whilst most people value their sleep, and increasingly want to work on achieving consistent and regular good sleep, few have proactively considered their actions pre-sleep and the impact they may have on their pending night's sleep.

So, what can a person do to ensure they get a good night's sleep regularly? How can they guarantee they're maximizing their ultimate (and free) performance enhancer – sleep? How can they help themselves to improve sleep and ultimately perform better in the workplace and deal with the demands of daily life? How can they regularly thrive in life with reliable optimal wellness? Below are some solutions which may help, but remember, sleep is entirely individualized. What works for one person may not work for another. Everyone's sleep requirement is different and, crucially, everyone's circumstances and ability to get good sleep are different.

> Socioeconomic factors in the world of sleep have a significant effect on sleep quality and quantity (Park *et al.*, 2021). Some people may experience bed poverty, as discussed in Chapter 7, or they may not have a spare room to escape to if their partner interrupts their sleep because of snoring or the logistics of shift work.
>
> Therefore, use the advice in this chapter to help your clients, but ensure it is applicable to them and be fully aware that the circumstances in relation to the opportunity to get good sleep will be different for each individual and may change over time.

When considering advising on sleep strategies, a good tip is to try one solution at a time, so your client understands what works for them. What helps them to relax to be in a good state to unwind and fall asleep is very much about what works for the individual. Attempting to change too many things at once may in fact cause poorer sleep, as the person must familiarize themselves with multiple changes to their sleep environment, routine and systems. Where sleep eludes a person over

STRATEGIES FOR GOOD SLEEP HEALTH

consecutive nights for half an hour or more, or they are frequently waking up and struggling to get back to sleep, then advise them to speak to their GP. If a client has a suspected sleep or circadian rhythm disorder, then practical strategies will not be the sole remedy, and they need to seek medical advice for diagnosis and appropriate treatment.

The first factor to identify when developing a strategy is to establish if there is something obvious preventing good sleep for the individual. For example, do they live in a noisy area where wearing earplugs may be beneficial? Or do they live in an area where there are bright lights outside their bedroom window, and so blackout blinds, curtains and a good eye mask may help with their sleep onset? Is there a temporary life stress or life phase that is upsetting sleep patterns, such as financial worries, a newborn baby or a new pet? These factors can be managed accordingly, and usually overcome in time, whilst adhering to some of the practical tips that follow.

SLEEP STRATEGY 1: SLEEP ROUTINE AND QUANTITY

It's good to reflect on a person's pre-sleep routine when discussing their sleep health. Query if they have ever considered their evening activities in relation to their effect on their ability to fall asleep? Do they think about, or even prioritize, what needs to be done ahead of bedtime each night? If the answer is 'no', then try to start to build a pre-sleep routine into their daily routine or plans. This is hard in a busy schedule, when factoring work commitments, family responsibilities and socializing into the equation often means a person's sleep (and general recovery needs) gets shunted down the priority list. Nonetheless, it's fundamental that sleep time is protected and personalized where possible (Espie, 2022a).

Aside from uncontrollable scenarios, such as young children waking in the night or illness, it's good to advise clients to aim to make the time before bed as consistent as possible. Having a consistent pre-sleep routine and time to bed will help to start to create good sleep practices. This will have an inevitable effect on achieving a regular get-up time, which is typically the 'anchor point' of the day as it is dictated somewhat by an individual's morning commitments, such as the commute to work and/ or family responsibilities. Regular bedtimes and get-up times also help with sleep onset and ensure sleep is maintained throughout the night, and ultimately aid a pathway to good sleep health. Having support from family members and employers for the demands of daily life can also help with a regular sleep routine.

I covered sleep quantity in Chapter 2, and you may remember that I described the general guidelines for optimal sleep quantity for a healthy adult, in the absence of a sleep or circadian rhythm disorder, being seven to nine hours per night. This is entirely individualized, however, as age, health, genetics and personal circumstances will affect how much sleep we need, but most healthy adults benefit from around this amount.

In terms of calculating time to bed, if an individual recognizes how much sleep they need, or at least can estimate it based on how alert they are during the day, then use their get-up time as the anchor point and calculate backwards to achieve the appropriate bedtime for them. For example, if they need eight hours' sleep and need be up at seven in the morning, then they should ensure their head is hitting the pillow by eleven in the evening. Having this as a simple strategy to sleep means they can mould and flex it around their working week to ensure sleep is optimal amid life's demands. Where this isn't always possible, they should aim for optimal sleep quantity for a realistic number of nights in the week and are therefore starting to establish a routine.

If people are pragmatic about their sleep schedule, then there is less pressure for it to become all-encompassing, and consequently, time to bed may not be a stressful time of the day. I have seen and heard from clients all too often who become anxious about their sleep schedule because they see it as a fixed point in time, without accounting for the fact that sometimes life is uncontrollable and chaotic. Being aware of needing a regular sleep schedule and adhering to it *as often as is possible* is preferable to attempting to maintain a rigid schedule every day and becoming stressed when this isn't realistic due to life pressures. An even worse scenario would be to be ignorant of the fact that a sleep schedule is important for physical and mental health.

As described in Chapter 2, your client can subjectively assess how much sleep they need simply by reviewing how they feel upon waking. If they can wake up without feeling overly groggy and are alert, fully refreshed and productive throughout the working day, then the likelihood is they are getting enough sleep. If not, then perhaps they need to adjust their sleep routine somewhat. Even adjusting bedtime by as little as 10–15 minutes will make a difference in terms of actual time asleep over a week, month and longer. Ultimately, this accumulation of improved sleep time will have long-term benefits for a person's physical and mental health.

Try to advise clients to use a traditional alarm clock for setting their get-up routine and, where possible, avoid using a smartphone as an alarm as these can potentially be a distraction pre-sleep. Many alarm clocks have a gradient setting which allows the user to set an alarm that builds up gradually, getting louder and louder until they turn it off. This means they get woken up progressively, rather than being 'bolted' awake. Other options may be to choose a sunrise alarm clock rather than a noisy alarm clock, which means a person wakes up more gradually and naturally. A sunrise alarm clock (or dawn simulation light) is an artificial light source that is integrated into a standard digital clock. It is timed to gradually wake a person at a selected time. Having gentler methods to wake up will place an individual in a much better place to start their day. Of course, this is not easy if they have small children jumping on the bed from the early hours most mornings, but you get the idea!

On the topic of alarm clocks, if a person is regularly sleeping well and has a good sleep routine, then it does raise the question of whether they need an alarm to wake them at all. Some argue that they like the 'safety net' of an alarm so they won't oversleep and miss an important morning schedule. You may have read that the British adventurer Bear Grylls made the rather tongue-in-cheek point about renaming the alarm clock to an 'opportunity clock' (Beecham, 2022), the idea being that it shouldn't be 'alarming' to be awake. Rather, an individual should wake up in a calm state and avoid any negative connotations of waking up. If an individual has had adequate sleep quality and quantity, they should therefore be refreshed and ready for the new day's opportunities. This kind of positive thinking and terminology is nothing new, but the approach to waking up as a positive experience, rather than being 'shocked' into a waking state, is perhaps something worth considering. If a person has had enough sleep and is feeling refreshed, then it could possibly be a good point to approach the start of the day with energy and positivity. Either way, an individual could choose a method or sound that wakes them softly, soothingly and steadily so they wake calmly and aren't 'surprised' into awakening.

Good sleep enhancement and management should be the primary aim of any strategy for a good night's sleep. However, sometimes sleep can get disrupted. This can often be predicted and therefore planned for accordingly – for example, an exam or a work trip. But one cannot always control nighttime sleep. Even if a person protects their sleep time, values and personalizes it and has a good strategy to sleep, sometimes they can't foresee when their sleep may be interrupted. For example, there may be illness or a temporary life stress, such as an emergency work problem. Therefore, there are times when an individual may need some help to combat the consequent sleepiness from restricted sleep, and this is where sleep extension can be beneficial.

SLEEP STRATEGY 2: SLEEP EXTENSION STRATEGIES

Sleep extension strategies, more commonly known as napping or sleep banking (Leger *et al.*, 2008; Mah *et al.*, 2011; Poussel *et al.*, 2015; Thornton *et al.*, 2016), are simple and easy measures to put in place. For starters, they're free and won't take long to achieve. They are particularly effective as, in general, they reduce the sleep pressure accumulated throughout the day and can be associated with improved nighttime sleep. This 'pressure' is the physiological drive that I described in Chapter 2, which an individual experiences when they are attempting to fall asleep. It naturally manifests at night; however, sleep pressure builds throughout the day and can feel quite strong typically in the afternoon nadir, approximately between two and four in the afternoon (Milner & Cote, 2009). This is when humans have a natural physiological 'dip' in their circadian rhythm and core body temperature reaches a low point. Typically, it is when people experience the post-lunch 'nodding donkey' feeling, and during this time is an ideal opportunity for a nap if it is safe and one has the motivation, opportunity and circumstances to do so (Gupta *et al.*, 2021).

Do bear in mind that the timing of naps should be considered wisely as incorrect timing may impact on nighttime sleep. The best timing for a nap varies according to an individual's sleep profile – that is, their personal 'sleep need'. The stability and timing of their sleep–wake schedules, their morningness–eveningness tendencies (chronotype), the quality of their sleep during the preceding night and their amount of prior wakefulness all account for their sleep need. Try not to advise a nap too close to the evening as this will have unintended consequences for nighttime sleep.

Fundamentally, sleep extension strategies fall into three main areas: prophylactic (where an individual may expect some sleep loss), replacement or compensatory naps (a reaction to a period of sleep loss) or appetitive (on demand), where an individual simply enjoys a nap and adds it into their day for convenience or enjoyment (Dinges, 1992; Gupta *et al.*, 2021). So, not all naps need to be in response to poor sleep.

To consider nap length, we need to refer to Chapter 2 and the advice around sleep cycles. You will recall the 90-minute sleep cycle with the four stages of sleep: light stages 1 and 2, stage 3 deep sleep and stage 4 dream sleep. Advise clients to maintain a nap length of between 20 and 30 minutes, or 90 minutes, so that they will be within the lighter sleep stages (stages 1 and 2) at the end of the nap, making waking easier than if in a deep sleep stage.

Generally, shorter naps will have a more immediate effect on reducing sleep pressure. Prolonged naps are also worthwhile, but the benefits take longer to gain any effect as the body must overcome a larger sleep inertia[1] (grogginess) upon waking (Milner & Cote, 2009). This is thought to mainly result from longer naps due to a higher likelihood of waking from slow-wave sleep or 'deep sleep'. Sleeping for 45–60 minutes generally means an individual would wake in stage 3 sleep (deep sleep). If they need to nap longer, then they should aim for 90 minutes, so they are more likely to wake in the transition from stage 4 sleep back to a lighter sleep stage, and therefore have less sleep inertia to overcome. In short, a person will wake less grumpy and groggy from a shorter nap than one lasting 45–60 minutes. Table 9.1 describes different nap lengths and their effects on an individual.

In terms of a person's motivation to nap, some people can fall asleep easily and enjoy a nap. Others feel they can 'muscle on through' daytime sleepiness, even if they do have the opportunity to nap. In these cases, it can be useful to advise an individual to try a 20-minute nap and see if they notice a difference over a few days. Possibly. Possibly not. Given the individual nature of sleep, naps aren't for everyone. The important point here is not to force a nap. If a person doesn't like napping, don't try to impose it on them. If they need it, have the opportunity and motivation to nap, and can do so safely, then it will naturally happen.

---

1   Sleep inertia is a reduced ability to think and perform upon awakening.

If your client doesn't enjoy napping, then some restful downtime will be equally beneficial for any recovery they may require. Other methods to aid wakefulness can also help with daytime sleepiness, for example, nutrition, hydration, physical activity and accessing daylight.

Table 9.1 Nap length and its effects

Nap length					
5 minutes	10 minutes	15 minutes	20 minutes	30+ minutes	< 90 minutes
Ultra-short nap No sleep inertia Minimal benefits Too short to have an effect	Short nap Limited to lighter stages of sleep (NREM) Minimal sleep inertia Easily awake and feel refreshed Concentration and response time improved Improvements last for approximately two hours	Significant benefits to alertness, concentration, focus and problem solving Some sleep inertia but overcome easily	Significant alert benefits Cognitive benefits quite great Learning capacity improved Memories consolidated Sleep inertia but can be overcome relatively easily	Restorative Improved mood state Helpful for memory consolidation Moving into deeper sleep stages Sleep inertia for up to 30 minutes post nap (sometimes more)	Full sleep cycle including REM sleep Helpful for emotional and procedural memory (technique learning) Wake more easily

In summary, proactive, reactive or simple enjoyment sleep extension strategies are incredibly useful, particularly for busy lifestyles. They can have a knock-on effect for improving nighttime sleep, hence the adage that 'sleep breeds sleep'. In terms of delivering daily performance at work and in general life, naps are a very effective way of regenerating for further tasks or stressors in the day, principally because they reduce, or offset, any sleep pressure a person may be experiencing. This allows the body to return to a state of balance and continue with the daily grind demanded of it. Bear in mind, though, that any intervention around sleep will be driven by an individual's sleep profile (their personal sleep need). How excessive an individual's daytime sleepiness is and their circumstances or opportunity to nap will also influence any sleep extension strategy (Milner & Cote, 2009).

A caveat to naps is that whilst inserting a nap into a weekly schedule is a simple means to promote good health and wellbeing, not everyone is partial to a nap and sometimes naps can be impractical or unsafe. Always ensure that the person can nap in a safe environment – for example, away from operating machinery and, if tired when driving, pulling over to sleep where it is safe to do so. The Royal Society for the Prevention of Accidents produced a road safety factsheet 'Driver fatigue and road collisions' with recommendations regarding driving if tired (ROSPA, 2024), and advised:

- Make sure you are fit to drive.
- Do not begin a journey if you are tired.
- Get sufficient sleep before embarking on a long journey.
- Avoid undertaking long journeys between midnight and 6 a.m., when natural alertness is at a minimum.
- Plan your journey to take sufficient breaks. A minimum break of at least 15 minutes after every two hours of driving is recommended. If you feel sleepy, stop in a safe place.
- Do not stop in an emergency refuge area or on the hard shoulder of a motorway.

Ultimately, naps are not always practical in busy working lives, but if you have a client who likes to nap and has the motivation, opportunity and circumstances to get a nap in at some point in the week, then they should aim to try it (Gupta *et al.* 2021). Enjoying a nap and trying to schedule one or two into a busy week may be the additional benefit to sleep and daytime functioning that a client has been looking for. They could start by adding one in where they can throughout the week and noticing if they feel different from doing so. This may then become part of their normal weekly routine as they embrace sleep as the ultimate, and free, performance enhancer.

These guidelines around napping assume that illness is not present. If the person is ill, they should sleep as much as they need to! If there is a potential sleep or circadian rhythm disorder which is causing excessive daytime sleepiness and therefore a lot of need for napping, then advise the person to seek advice from their GP.

SLEEP STRATEGY 3: SLEEP SYSTEMS

The term 'sleep system' sounds quite technical for something that is supposed to be relaxing and help you sleep, but essentially a sleep system is a person's bedroom, bed, pillow, bedding, mattress and bed clothing. There are numerous different options out there for having a good sleep system, and given the fact that humans spend a third of their lives asleep, it's worth investing in one that works for the individual, has some longevity and provides them with the comfort and support they need to get a healthy night's sleep. Bed Advice UK, part of the National Bed Federation, have some sensible and practical tips available on their websites for buying beds and mattresses, and are signposted at the end of this book.

Bedframes and mattresses

You can't put a price on good quality and quantity of sleep. The bed itself should suit the individual's comfort needs. Cost is obviously an issue for some people, but I try to advise people to spend what they can afford and consider the fact that for a £1000 bed, shared with a partner over seven years, the cost is 40 pence per night, so investing in a good bed can be quite cost effective (National Bed Federation, 2020). Of course, not everyone is able to do this and, as I have already alluded to, bed poverty is a concerning issue.

Where possible, individuals should 'try before they buy' a bed. If buying online, ensure there is a grace period where the bed can be returned if it hasn't met expectations. Importantly, advise clients to ensure the bed is built to industry standards, so is safe (e.g. look for the National Bed Federation 'tick' for quality assurance) and clean.

With regard to the size of bed, the bigger the better, where bedroom space allows. More actual space in the bed to sleep means less disturbance and therefore better quality and quantity of sleep. Whether people share a bed with a partner or get it all to themselves is a factor in how well they sleep, and partner disturbance is one of the most common reported contributors to poor sleep.

The social aspect of sleep has received limited focus in sleep science literature, but it has been reported that approximately 60 per cent of adults have a bed partner (Walker, 2024c). Minor movements of the body can occur during normal, healthy sleep, and by how much is down to the individual, although men do tend to move around more than women (Pankhurst & Home, 1994; Skarpsno *et al.*, 2017). Of course, some people don't share a bed, but either way, sleep quality and quantity are individualized, so getting a sleep system that is comfortable for the individual is important.

> You may have read recent reports around the 'sleep divorce', 'sleep separation' or unconventional and alternative sleep arrangements. This is where couples consciously choose to sleep either in separate bedrooms or separate beds to aid their sleep quality and quantity. It is a personal choice with added benefits and pitfalls depending on the reason for the separation. Sometimes a person may need to improve their sleep for reasons of mental health. Alternatively, it may be a more simple or practical reason such as that their bed partner moves a lot in the night or they are using a CPAP intervention. Sleeping separately may affect personal relations too, or improve them(!), but this is a private matter which a client may or may not wish to divulge.

The standard double bed (135 cm x 190 cm or 4 ft 6 in x 6 ft 3 in) is the typical choice in the UK. Unfortunately, this doesn't offer much sleep space, with only 70 centimetres (2 ft 3 in) of space for each person. If you consider the fact that by the time a person is 50 years old, they would have spent approximately the equivalent of 16 years asleep, it's worth investing, where possible, in a good, large bed.

Obviously, a bed needs a mattress, and choosing one can be daunting with so many options out there. Yet it's important to recognize how something as seemingly trivial as a mattress could significantly impact a good night's sleep. In one year, a person would spend approximately 3000 hours (over 120 days) in bed, and in just a seven-year period a mattress will undergo 20,000 hours of wear and tear, so getting the right mattress for a person should be a priority. In fact, it's recommended that a mattress is replaced every ten years. Not everyone will be able to commit to this, but where possible, it's good to aim to do so.

Specifying a person's ideal mattress is extremely subjective as everyone will have their own idea of the perfect mattress in terms of firmness, height, spring and temperature. They may also need a hypoallergenic mattress and bed linen to alleviate any hypersensitivity or allergy symptoms which could disturb sleep. Mattress comfort can also be determined by sleeping position and body mass, and cost plays a part too.

Advise clients to take the time to decide on a mattress, as uncomfortable sleep systems can lead to additional issues such as musculoskeletal pain, and therefore a restless night's sleep. Sounds simple, but also recommend that clients ensure the base of the bed and the mattress size match. You'd be amazed how many times this isn't the case! Compatible bed and mattress size means greater comfort and better sleep.

Safety is important too, so advise your clients to ensure their mattress has a fire label sewn in that refers to BS7177, the British safety specification for resistance to ignition of mattresses, divans and bed bases (Bed Advice UK, 2024). Also, direct clients to look for the National Bed Federation (NBF) tick label. The 'Made by an approved NBF member' label is given to NBF-approved products that have undergone thorough independent reviews. This verifies that they comply with strict regulations on flammability, cleanliness of fillings and trade descriptions, and meet other important legal requirements relating to the manufacture of their products (Bed Advice UK, 2024). Always advise your clients that they should buy from a bed brand that has been NBF approved as this provides quality assurance and a safety guarantee of the product.

Bedding and pillows

Bed linen is also an important part of the sleep system. This includes the duvet, bed sheets, pillowcases and blankets.

The Thermal Overall Grade (tog) is an indicator of how warm a duvet is. This rating is based on a calculation completed under laboratory conditions rather than an actual life scenario, so should only be taken as a guide. Remember also that there are other factors that will influence how comfortable a person finds their bedding, not least personal comfort and body temperature.

Generally, tog ratings increase in increments of 1.5, with the lowest tog rating being 1–3 (very cool), whilst the highest generally available is 15 (very warm). Table 9.2 provides a guide as to the duvet tog and season and the relative warmth feel. Although how a person perceives their duvet is totally subjective, it is useful to have a guide.

Duvets can have a variety of fillings, the most common being goose down or duck feather, with different fillings providing varying levels of warmth. Therefore, a light, thin duvet is not always a cool duvet. As a general guide, advise clients to ensure the duvet tog is suitable for the season, not too high for the summer, yet warm enough for the winter.

Table 9.2 Duvet tog guide and seasons (DuvetAdvisor, n.d.)

Duvet season	Equivalent TOG	Warmth feel
High summer/summer	4.5 or less	Light and cool
Spring and autumn	7–9 tog	Cool to moderate
Spring, autumn and winter	10.5 tog	Warm
Winter	13.5 tog	Very warm
All year/all seasons duvet	All seasons duvet 4.5 + 9 tog = 13.5 tog	A combination duvet allowing one to be cool, warm or very warm
Partner duvet	Twin/partner/his and hers duvet Often a 9 tog and a 4 tog	Warmer on one half, cooler on the other

Believe it or not, duvets do exist for differing needs of bed partners. The Scandinavian sleep method has received some popularity of late (thank you, TikTok) and there may be some benefits to it. This method involves couples using two separate duvets to minimize sleep disruption. Partners can still share a bed but have individual single-size duvets. Not only is this more economical than buying two separate beds, but it offers sleep personalization at a whole new level and prevents war of the duvet. Partner duvets are also available where one duvet is separated down the middle with a different tog rating for each side. Mattresses can also be purchased with a different firmness on each side. Whilst the Scandinavian sleep method won't fix all sleep problems, it may help with a few.

For women experiencing sleep disturbances related to menstrual cycle, pregnancy, postpartum or the menopause transition symptoms, separate duvets could be of great benefit, particularly in relation to body temperature. Having freedom over their temperature whilst sleeping, whether a hot sleeper or someone more on the cool side, and without having to impact or consult with their bed partner could be a significant help for a woman experiencing sleep disturbances throughout her lifetime (Pacheco, 2023). For example, if hot flushes are common, having a personal duvet allows a woman to adjust her thermal comfort as required during the night. Equally, a woman enduring restless sleep with pregnancy symptoms may be relieved to have her own duvet so as not to keep waking her bed partner whilst trying to get comfortable throughout the night.

Regarding pillows, to avoid any musculoskeletal issues relating to a person's sleeping position, advise clients not to have too many pillows to ensure the musculoskeletal alignment of the head, neck and spine. Make sure pillows are comfortable for the individual and, if needed, hypoallergenic. Ideally, choose a pillow based on its thickness (loft), firmness, support, shape, material composition and, of course, price.

Personalized comfort for sleeping also depends on whether a person is a side, front or back sleeper. If a side sleeper, as most people are (Skarpsno *et al.*, 2017), advise them to try to use a pillow to prevent the hips from rolling forward in sleep in order to maintain a neutral spine. Also, if a person is a side sleeper, consider a pillow's 'loft' as they will need more cushioning between their head and neck. This may be relevant if, for example, a woman is pregnant and requires a pregnancy pillow to ease discomfort during the night when sleeping on her side.

The material type of bed linen is also important for sleep comfort. For example, cotton is breathable and therefore better than silk bed-sheets for keeping cool. This part of the sleep system can be very relevant for a women's sleep; cool linen sheets may be useful, for example, if a woman is experiencing hot flushes, or it may be they require a warm duvet for being up in the night for night feeds with a newborn.

There are many choices out there for all aspects of a sleep system; advise clients to seek out the 'try before you buy' options if they can. Also, from a general hygiene point of view, ensure bed linen (and clothing) is washed regularly and, if possible, get a mattress topper for additional comfort.

Finally, don't overlook the fact that, as mentioned in Chapter 7, bed poverty is a huge issue in the UK (and wider global society). If you think a client needs support in this area, there are signposts at the end of this book.

Sleepwear

What a person wears to bed will influence body comfort and temperature. To fall asleep, an individual needs to feel cool, but what they wear is their choice. Breathable, light cotton clothing is best for sleeping in, but it's all down to personal preference. A survey in 2018 of 1200 UK adults revealed some interesting findings with regard to nightwear choices. Most people surveyed preferred to sleep naked, or in underwear or pyjamas, but a small percentage reported sleeping in hoodies, tracksuits or onesies (Dillner, 2017). The latter sound hot and uncomfortable to me, but sleep is individualized!

The advantage of sleeping unclothed, or in underwear, is that the body is cooler, and humans need to feel cool to trigger the onset of sleep. Sometimes wearing underwear can cause issues, particularly in women, where wearing tight underwear overnight may affect the sensitive areas around the vulva, leading to vaginal infections such as thrush.[2] Overall, nighttime clothing that makes a person feel hot is unlikely to help them sleep and won't be a wise choice if they are also experiencing body temperature fluctuations.

What a woman sleeps in influences nighttime comfort levels, but may change throughout the month or year, never mind the phase of life they are in. For women who experience excessive symptoms in different phases of their life, such as heavy menstrual flow or night sweats, having a change of clothes to hand overnight may be useful to help return to sleep. Similarly, if a woman is breastfeeding, then investing in comfortable bed clothing that allows them to feed easily and means they can get back to sleep as quickly as possible after feeding is worthwhile.

There is no health benefit to what to wear for sleep – it's a personal choice and only limited by temperature. The bottom line (no pun intended) is for an individual to wear what they're comfortable in and make sure it is light, breathable and loose-fitting. So wearing pyjamas or sleeping as nature intended is really up to the individual (I'd advise against the tracksuits and onesies though!).

As a summary, the headlines for sleep systems are:

- Research before buying a bed. Try out beds, mattresses and pillows in a shop, if possible, and look at the reviews. Online purchases often offer a trial before committing to buying, so this may also be a useful option.

---

2   Thrush is a common yeast infection that affects men and women. It's usually harmless, but it can be uncomfortable and keep returning. Refer to a GP if thrush is suspected.

- Wear comfortable, breathable clothing.
- Change a mattress every ten years if able to do so.
- Ensure bedding is appropriate for the season.
- Ensure bedding allows good musculoskeletal alignment of head, neck and back.
- Buy as big a bed as is practically possible.

SLEEP STRATEGY 4: SLEEP ENVIRONMENT

Whilst sleep systems are important, having the ideal bedroom environment is paramount since the bedroom plays host to the beginning and end of daily activities and assists in preparation for and recovery from these activities (Van Deun *et al.*, 2015).

Room temperature

To aid sleep onset, humans need a cool, calm and dimly lit environment. Bedroom temperature is important as core body temperature in humans has its own circadian rhythm (as described for sleep in Chapter 2) and decreases during the evening and to its lowest point during the night. This decrease is associated with the onset of sleep, so too warm an environment will not aid sleep. Therefore, advise your clients to try to ensure a neutral bedroom temperature to help the onset and maintenance of sleep. It is down to individual preference, but ideally, not too hot or cold, typically 18–20°C.

I usually recommend that people plan their bedroom environment to help with sleep onset. For example, if the room is known to be warm, then use strategies to cool the room before sleep (e.g. lower air conditioning, open a window or use a fan). Also, warming the skin will help core body temperature fall to what is needed for sleep onset, so having a warm bath before bed can potentially help. Equally, if the room is too cold, then have a blanket or hot water bottle to hand to help find a comfortable temperature to sleep in.

Light and noise considerations

Previously, it was thought that human circadian rhythms were insensitive to light and more receptive to social cues for circadian rhythm entrainment (Duffy & Czeisler, 2009). However, it became widely accepted that cells in the eye (photoreceptors) are sensitive to light and dark, and ultimately communicate with areas in the brain to signal to us if it is night or daytime, and therefore time to go to sleep or wake up.

As described in Chapter 2, the process of informing the body of a sleep or wake state involves a complex interaction of photic (light) information which passes from the retina (the light-sensitive tissue layer of our eye), through the retinohypothalamic tract, deep into the brain to the hypothalamus.[3] This houses the suprachiasmatic nucleus (SCN), which signals to other areas of the brain to start the process of falling asleep or remain alert and awake, primarily by instructing the pineal gland to press 'go' on melatonin release or not. As you may recall, in Chapter 2 we talked about melatonin release being linked to the light–dark cycle and being a signaller of sleep or wake. As our sleep–wake rhythm interacts with the light–dark cycle, melatonin is either released or supressed, depending on whether it is light or dark. Daylight, therefore, is crucial to our daily rhythmic routine and our nighttime sleep (Wirz-Justice, Skene & Münch, 2021).

The sleep scientist Professor Matthew Walker has spoken about 'junk light' where humans are exposed to excessive electrical light in the evening – for example, city living where bright lights are effectively on 24/7 (Walker, 2024b). This delays the release of the hormone melatonin, which delays sleep onset and therefore decreases quality and quantity. Where possible, recommend that clients try to minimize exposure to bright light in the home in the evenings.

BLUE LIGHT THEORY

Light acts on the body by two pathways. First, what you can see and, therefore, do as a result (visual perception, responses and reflexes) are governed by the primary optic tract (a pathway from your eye to the brain). The second pathway is the retinohypothalamic tract – the pathway from our eye to the hypothalamus – which has a role in sleep regulation (Holzman, 2010).

Visible light has many wavelengths to it (measured in nanometres) and consists of a spectrum of different colours – remember the prism

---

3   The hypothalamus is an area deep in the brain that governs our circadian (body clock), endocrine (hormones) and neural-behavioural functions (nervous system and behaviour).

of light from school physics lessons? It is the brain that tells us that visible light is white, although other colours in the white light spectrum (400–700 nm) can be detected by cells in our retina. One in particular is blue light wavelengths (450–495 nm), which can potentially play a part in overall sleep health.

Smartphones, laptops and other devices that emit blue light have traditionally been associated with sleep restriction. Blue light stimulates the brain to increase the release of serotonin (a neurotransmitter) and suppresses melatonin release, which delays sleep onset. However, recent studies have questioned whether the strength of blue light emitted from such devices is strong enough to suppress melatonin production sufficiently to affect nighttime sleep (Bauducco et al., 2024). Therefore, the need to avoid blue light before sleep may after all be a 'sleep myth' (Gradisar, 2024). This is quite a turnaround in the sleep science literature, which has previously emphasized the damaging effect of blue light on melatonin secretion.

However, sleep onset, and ultimately sleep quality and quantity, may still be affected by what people watch or play on their devices through the cognitive arousal such devices bring. Certainly, heightened cognitive arousal at night is linked to objective sleep disturbances and indicators of physiological hyperarousal at night and during the day (Kalmbach et al., 2020).

Whilst downtime for a lot of people involves watching television or playing a computer game, it is important to be aware of how this can affect sleep onset. Watching a programme may in fact relax someone, but having the will to turn it off at the desired time for sleep is vital for successful sleep onset. For example, if an individual does watch television, then ideally they should watch something mundane, at a lower volume than usual, and perhaps something they have seen before. If the latest TV drama instils feelings of anxiety and thrill-seeking late at night, then they are likely to be awake for longer than they should be. Having a level of self-awareness and being rigorous with turning off devices at the preferred sleep time and therefore avoiding going beyond this critical time point is fundamental to healthy sleep.

Excessive noise can also affect the sleep environment. Where possible, advise clients to avoid having devices on too loud in the bedroom and to listen to soft, calming music or have the radio or television on at a lower volume if that is a part of their sleep strategy. If they live in a noisy area, maybe try earplugs or an eye mask (refer to the section 'Eye masks and ear plugs' under 'Sleep strategy 7: Sleep aids').

In summary, ideally the sleep environment needs to be cool, calm and dimly lit. It is entirely an individual's preference as to how this may be achieved, but certainly a loud, noisy, warm environment won't be conducive to good sleep.

SLEEP STRATEGY 5: NUTRITION

Nutrition and sleep have a reciprocal relationship in the same way mental health and sleep (Chapter 7) and physical activity and sleep do (more on this later in this chapter). Studies report that diets rich in fibre, whole grains, fruit and vegetables are associated with longer sleep duration, better sleep quality and fewer insomnia symptoms (Zuraikat & St-Onge, 2020). Equally, it is well documented that insufficient sleep negatively impacts on dietary intake (Zuraikat *et al.*, 2021).

Nutrition and sleep can encompass many factors, including the type of food a person eats, the timing of meals and the amount of food ingested. This section provides some information around meal timings and good food and drink practices for good sleep, along with a few suggestions for foods that may indeed aid sleep. For more detailed resources, do advise clients to seek guidance from a qualified dietitian or nutritionist. Recommendations for suitably qualified practitioners are available in the resources section at the end of this book.

There are particular nutrition strategies that a person could use to help get a good night's sleep. For example, certain foods contain the essential amino acid tryptophan.[4] This is not made in the body but ingested exogenously. It is important for sleep as it helps to make serotonin, a neurotransmitter which, as mentioned in Chapter 2, is useful in the communication pathways of the sleep–wake cycle, particularly with melatonin. Foods containing tryptophan include high-protein foods such as chicken, eggs, cheese, fish, peanuts, pumpkin and sesame seeds, leafy greens, watercress, broccoli, milk, turkey, tofu and soy. The

---

4   Amino acids are the building blocks of proteins. They also serve as precursors for other body compounds such as hormones and neurotransmitters.

recommended daily intake of tryptophan is 4 mg per kilogram of body weight. So, for example, a glass of warm milk before bed, or during the night if one can't sleep, may help sleep onset. Other foods that may help with sleep onset and maintenance are kiwi fruit (packed with serotonin) or tart cherry juice (contains melatonin). For more detailed information on foods that can aid sleep, refer to the available literature (Pereira *et al.*, 2020; Cheon & Kim, 2022).

In addition to the light–dark cycle, mealtimes are another robust rhythm that the body uses to synchronize itself to the daily 24-hour cycle. Certain energy metabolism- and appetite-regulating hormones, such as insulin (glucose metabolism), leptin (appetite) and ghrelin (hunger), follow circadian rhythms which, when disrupted, could lead to serious metabolic consequences (Boege *et al.*, 2021). Therefore, mealtimes should be at the appropriate time of day, to help with body homeostasis and avoid any desynchronization of physiological processes.

Evidence suggests that eating late into the evening before bed can have an adverse effect on positive energy balance and lead to increases in body mass. This has a concomitant effect on the prevalence of cardiometabolic disease, such as heart attacks, strokes or type 2 diabetes (Boege *et al.*, 2021).

To be able to fall asleep easily, the timing of meals is important. Studies are scarce, but overall, mealtimes too close to bedtime have been associated with a prolonged sleep onset latency (time from lights out to falling asleep), indicating a difficulty in sleep onset (Yasuda, Kishi & Fujita, 2023). Other cofounding factors preventing a short sleep onset latency may also come into play, such as a mental health issue or a physical comorbidity, but ideally mealtimes less than two hours before sleep should be discouraged.

Equally, how much or how little a person eats can upset sleep quality and quantity. Consuming too much food before bedtime can lead to discomfort, indigestion and heartburn, all of which disrupt one's ability to fall and stay asleep. Conversely, not consuming enough food before bed can cause one to feel hungry, which also has a negative effect on sleep (Aggeler, 2024).

In terms of hydration, drinking enough water throughout the day is critical to health. Ideally, healthy adults should aim to drink approximately two litres of water per day (British Dietetics Association, 2023), although fitness level, environment and gender all influence how much fluid a person requires. As a general guide, you could advise clients to use morning urine colour to indicate hydration status, with a pale-yellow colour suggesting good hydration.

It's also recommended to avoid drinking too close to bedtime as this may cause an individual to need numerous trips to the bathroom throughout the night. It's normal to get up once or twice during the night to use the bathroom, but any more than that interrupts sleep by quite a bit, so advise clients to back off the fluid intake an hour or two before bedtime. If excessive urination symptoms persist, even after reducing fluid intake, then advise clients to talk to their GP.

Caffeine

Certain foods and drinks will have a negative effect on sleep, and none more so than caffeine. It is widely used in foods and beverages for its stimulating and alertness-promoting effects. There are many variations in caffeinated products, including chocolate, energy drinks and tea, but coffee is the most potent. Table 9.3 gives an indication of the caffeine content in different beverages.

Table 9.3 Caffeine content of different beverages (Pacheco & Cotliar, 2024)

Beverage	Caffeine content (mg)
227 ml (8 oz) cup of coffee	95–200 mg
227 ml (8 oz) energy drink	70–100 mg
227 ml (8 oz) cup of tea	14–60 mg

Generally, caffeine can impair the onset and maintenance of subsequent sleep. It reduces total sleep time, sleep efficiency, sleep intensity and satisfaction levels, and increases sleep onset latency and wake after sleep onset (Weibel et al., 2021; Gardiner et al., 2023). It is a common sleep robber in that it influences the chemical pathways involved in the sleep pressure build-up and essentially blunts the sleep-promoting centre from taking over from the arousal centre at the point at which a person would normally 'flip-flop' between the two states (as described in Chapter 2).

With caffeine intake, the central nervous system becomes stimulated, causing a state of alertness, the opposite state of where a person needs to be for sleep onset. However, in some cases when caffeine is continuously consumed throughout the day, daily caffeine intake has been shown to have less of an effect than acute consumption (Weibel *et al.*, 2021).

The maximum amount of caffeine advised for a person is 400 mg per day and it has a half-life[5] of approximately two to 12 hours, meaning it can stay in the body for a relatively short time or for a while (Pacheco & Cotliar, 2024). This can vary from person to person, and some people can tolerate caffeine better than others in terms of its effect on subsequent sleep. The wide range in the half-life of caffeine indicates the fact that many factors influence how a person metabolizes caffeine – for example, body mass and hydration status (Pacheco & Cotliar, 2024).

> Overuse of caffeine may lead to insomnia symptoms or worsen pre-existing insomnia. Consuming it with the purpose of staying awake at night may lead to headaches, excessive daytime sleepiness, anxiety, frequent nighttime wakenings and overall poorer sleep quality. Caffeine-interrupted sleep can lead to restricted sleep and the associated issues – for example, fatigue and problems with learning, memory, problem-solving and regulation of emotions.

I would advise your clients that if they like drinks containing caffeine and they tolerate it well, then having the odd caffeinated drink won't affect their sleep too much. General guidelines around caffeine consumption are that if a person enjoys it and can tolerate it, they should front-load caffeine intake at the start of the day and reduce it from lunchtime onwards by switching to decaffeinated drinks, water or fruit or herbal tea. If a client is particularly susceptible to caffeine and they find even small amounts affect subsequent nighttime sleep, then it may be best they avoid it wherever possible. Like most activities related to sleep, caffeine ingestion is a personal choice, unless advised by a medic not to ingest it at all.

---

5   Half-life is the time it takes for the concentration of a substance such as caffeine to fall to half of its initial value.

Alcohol

Another common substance that can have a detrimental effect on sleep is, unsurprisingly, alcohol, which has worryingly unfavourable consequences for sleep, even in small quantities.

Many people use alcohol as a strategy to help them get to sleep and drinking an evening tipple can be a regular part of their life. The Sleep Council's *Great British Bedtime Report* (2017) reported that 25 per cent of those questioned used alcohol to help them nod off (an increase from 16 per cent in 2013).

So why is it used in this way? Primarily, it is seen as a means to wind down and relax of an evening. It is a central nervous system depressant that causes brain activity to slow down, thus reducing alertness, even when drunk in small quantities. Essentially, it has a sedative effect that switches off brain cell activity as sleep onset beckons, making one feel relaxed and sleepy (Park *et al.*, 2015), but the consumption of alcohol, especially in excess, has been linked to poor sleep quality and quantity. So, whilst your clients may think that alcohol might help them get off to sleep quickly, that odd glass of wine or two, beer, or gin and tonic can play havoc with their sleep quality, and quantity, and drinking alcohol to aid sleep is not a good habit to get into.

Alcohol is a major culprit for disrupting a night's sleep as it can interfere with the body's chemical processes needed for sound sleep. How does this happen? Alcohol effectively fragments sleep, making it more restless and less restorative. Increased wakenings in the latter half of the night, when the alcohol's relaxing effect wears off, prevent an individual from achieving the required sleep quality from deep NREM (stage 3) and REM (stage 4) sleep. As the night progresses, this can create an imbalance in sleep architecture, with REM sleep in particular being affected, with decreased overall sleep quality, shorter sleep duration and more sleep disruptions (Bryan & Singh, 2024).

The REM stage of sleep (stage 4 sleep or the 'dream sleep' phase), as you may recall from Chapter 2, is a critical stage of sleep for numerous aspects of health and wellness, including learning and memory, creativity and, importantly, rebalancing moods and emotions. As sleep progresses throughout the night, alcohol delays and limits REM sleep, meaning the aspect of sleep architecture that helps emotional regulation is reduced. The delayed onset of the first REM sleep period occurs with all doses of alcohol and appears to be the most recognizable effect of alcohol on REM sleep, followed by the reduction in total night REM sleep (Bryan & Singh, 2024). It isn't large amounts of alcohol that cause these alterations to sleep architecture either. The alterations to the REM sleep stage have consequences for daytime functioning in terms of emotional control and coping mechanisms. Later in the night, once any alcohol ingested has been metabolized, there is an increased likelihood of stage 1 sleep, the lightest stage of sleep. This leads to frequent nighttime awakenings, fragmented, poor-quality sleep and early morning wakefulness.

Alcohol is also a diuretic, meaning it will increase the body's production of urine. It does so by preventing the brain from releasing an important hormone (vasopressin) that regulates the amount of water in the body. The diuretic effect sends a person running to the loo more often, perhaps upsetting sleep, and dehydrates the body as it encourages too much water to be dispersed out of the body. This puts the body under strain and can lead to headaches, which may also prevent sleep onset. The associated consequences of dehydration making a person feel hot, thirsty and generally uncomfortable will also contribute to increased night wakenings and overall poorer sleep quality.

Whilst drinking in moderation is generally considered safe, how an individual reacts to alcohol can vary, so its impact on sleep largely depends on the individual. Table 9.4 shows, quite alarmingly, how much sleep is affected by different amounts of alcohol intake. For women, less than one drink can affect sleep quality and quantity by nearly 10 per cent, and more than one drink by as much as nearly 40 per cent (Bryan & Singh, 2024).

Table 9.4 How will alcohol affect sleep? (Bryan & Singh, 2024)

Amount	Effect on sleep
Low Less than 2 drinks for men and 1 drink for women	Sleep quality decreased by 9.3%
Moderate Approximately 2 drinks for men and 1 drink for women	Sleep quality decreased by 24%
High More than 2 drinks for men and 1 drink for women	Sleep quality decreased by 39.2%

Another disadvantage of alcohol in relation to sleep is that an individual can develop a tolerance for alcohol quite quickly, leading them to drink more before bed in order to help them initiate sleep. The sleep-inducing effects of alcohol reduce with more consumption, and the subsequent sleep disruption resulting from alcohol use may lead to more daytime fatigue and sleepiness. A Catch-22 scenario arises, with more alcohol consumed to aid sleep, but poorer sleep as a result of the increased alcohol consumption. This has become quite a hot topic in my female health and sleep webinars, with women commenting on the negative effects of alcohol on how they feel they are thriving on a daily basis or in life in general, and their associated quality of sleep.

Unfortunately, there is also a link between long-term alcohol abuse and chronic sleep problems. People with alcohol use disorders commonly experience insomnia symptoms, and studies have shown that alcohol use can exacerbate the symptoms of sleep apnoea, the condition where an individual takes in too little oxygen whilst asleep, resulting in many bouts of light sleep, with wakings after sleep onset and very little deep-stage sleep (Bryan & Singh, 2024). In these instances, it is best to recommend that someone seeks help from either their GP or some of the resources signposted at the end of this book.

The good news is that if an individual stops consuming alcohol pre-sleep, they can return to healthy sleep in time as there is a gradual improvement in sleep once alcohol has been taken out of the equation. Immediate benefits are minimal, however, as the body must readjust to the absence of alcohol. Sleep remains a challenge with increased sleep disturbances and alcohol withdrawal symptoms, such as anxiety, restlessness and night sweats. An individual may also experience vivid dreams or nightmares as REM sleep begins to return to its normal proportion of the 90-minute sleep cycle (REM rebound). There are some subtle initial indicators of sleep improvement during the immediate phase of alcohol withdrawal, though, as it becomes easier to fall asleep naturally and there may be fewer nighttime awakenings (Neurolaunch, 2024). Up until approximately 12 weeks after cessation of alcohol consumption, there are more notable improvements in a person's sleep. There is a gradual increase in sleep duration and quality, and an improvement in the ability to fall asleep naturally and stay asleep throughout the night. As time progresses, there is a more profound normalization of sleep patterns, with the circadian rhythm becoming more synchronized to light–dark cycles and an enhancement of normal sleep architecture with NREM stage 3 and REM sleep stages. Ther is also a reduction in sleep-related anxiety and insomnia symptoms. After approximately 12 weeks, there is a full restoration of the natural sleep–wake cycle, with an established circadian rhythm making it easier to fall asleep and wake up at consistent times. There is, therefore, more regularity in sleep patterns, equating to better sleep quality and daytime functioning. Overall, quality of life is improved with increased daytime energy levels, better mood and enhanced cognitive function (Neurolaunch, 2024).

Generally, an individual will experience fragmented, less restorative rest following pre-sleep alcohol consumption. If a client is regularly consuming alcohol to help them fall asleep, then it's probably a good idea to advise them to try something else that makes them feel relaxed pre-sleep, as per some of the practical relaxation strategies provided in the section 'Sleep strategy 8: Relaxation techniques' below. Other recommendations would be to try to swap the evening tipple for either a herbal tea or milky drink, which will help with relaxation and preparing the body for sleep.

In summary, people should aim to develop a bedtime routine or ritual that does not involve alcohol on too regular a basis. The aim is to create an almost unconscious association between bedtime and the sensations of drifting off to sleep. My recommendations aren't not to drink alcohol, more to recognize that alcohol consumption is a personal choice that a client should make whilst being informed that it does negatively influence their sleep. If you suspect a client has a more serious connection to alcohol, then further support for alcohol misuse is available through organizations such as Alcohol Change, a GP and other places listed in the resources section at the end of this book.

Supplements

There is a myriad of supplements reported to aid sleep. I am not a qualified dietitian or nutritionist so I am not about to delve in great technical detail into the benefits or drawbacks of supplements in relation to sleep, but I do feel duty-bound to make a salient point about supplement use, particularly for those readers who are supporting athletes.

Importantly, if a client is on any prescribed medication, I would advise they check with their GP before taking any form of supplement. It goes without saying that practitioners working with athletes should follow the advice from the World Anti-Doping Agency (WADA) and their respective local anti-doping agency (e.g. in the UK we have UK Anti-Doping (UKAD)), and that athletes should follow a 'food first' principle when starting out on their sporting career. As the athletes develop,

STRATEGIES FOR GOOD SLEEP HEALTH

and maybe become part of a UK Sport-funded World Class Development or World Class Performance Programme, or involved in a professional sport, supplements may be something they ask about with regard to aiding sleep (or for a wider issue, but that's not for this book to focus on).

> Following the principle of strict liability – that is, athletes are solely responsible for any banned substance they use, attempt to use, or is found in their system, regardless of how it got there or whether there was any intention to cheat (World Anti-Doping Agency, 2021) – athletes should be careful around using supplements in general. In the context of this book, I will focus on supplements purporting to aid sleep.

UK Anti Doping advise that athletes must always 'assess the need, assess the risk and assess the consequences' when it comes to considering taking any form of supplement (UKAD, 2023). Everyone, including athlete support personnel (ASP), has a duty to protect clean sport. Anti-doping regulations apply to ASP too, so if you are a practitioner supporting athletes, ensuring that you are educated about anti-doping practices is key to supporting clients in the sporting world. More information on anti-doping education can be found on the WADA and UKAD websites, signposted at the end of this book.

Practitioners should ensure athletes can make an informed choice regarding supplement use for aiding sleep and that athletes *always* check supplements on the website Informed Sport (www.informedsport.com) before using one. This is a global testing and certification programme for sports and nutritional supplements. Whilst this website doesn't offer an absolute guarantee of the safety of a supplement, it does show details of batch-tested supplements in terms of whether they are banned in or out of competition. I would urge practitioners to advise athletes on other strategies to aid sleep before recommending the supplement route.

Supplements in general have the least amount of scientific evidence from studies documenting their pros and cons in relation to sleep. Supplements are not formal medications,[6] and therefore not subjected

---

6   Athletes can also check medications on the website Global Dro (www.globaldro. com).

to the same rigorous trials as prescribed medications. Consequently, there is considerably less oversight of sleep aids sold as dietary supplements compared to prescription medicines, which do require clinical governance.

There is also a huge diversity in available sleep supplements, and brands can create sleep aids made of just one ingredient or a blend a few together, without the need for any legislation. Most sleep supplements market themselves on their calming effects and it may be that they potentially offer some anxiolytic (anxiety-relieving) properties – for example, valerian root, chamomile and lavender. However, when advising clients, I would refer them to a qualified dietitian or nutritionist to help them make an informed and safe choice around their supplement use. I would also educate them about other practical strategies to aid their sleep that may be of benefit, before parting with their cash on supplements which may or may not have a positive effect on sleep.

Melatonin supplementation receives quite a lot of attention in the media, and research suggests it has a positive effect on sleep in some adults (Fatemeh *et al.*, 2022). Prescribed melatonin to aid sleep stems from clinical work supporting families of children with conditions such as autism spectrum disorder (ASD) and attention deficit hyperactivity disorder (ADHD), where it may improve total sleep time, sleep onset latency and sleep efficiency (Nogueira *et al.*, 2023). It has also been reported as having benefits in helping overcome jet lag (Herxheimer *et al.*, 2002) and is one of the most common forms of self-medication for sleep and jet lag (Halson, Burke & Pearce, 2019). However, with varied findings observed in the studies conducted, the actual benefit to total sleep time from melatonin supplementation is up for debate (Fatemeh *et al.*, 2022).

Further, the regulation and availability of melatonin differs across countries. It is considered a medication in countries such as the UK, some parts of Europe, Australia and New Zealand, and is available on prescription only, typically for the aforementioned spectrum disorders or where a patient has a circadian rhythm disorder. It is not illegal to be in possession of melatonin in the United States, however, where it is accessible as an over-the-counter non-prescription supplement, and therefore unregulated (Halson *et al.*, 2019).

Unfortunately, melatonin supplementation can create a dependency and other side effects, such as dizziness, headaches and nausea (Garcia,

2020). For clients interested in melatonin supplementation, I would advise trying some of the practical strategies suggested in this chapter first, and if there is a clinical need for a prescription, then they need to speak to their GP.

For more detailed information regarding nutrition and sleep, please do get advice from a qualified dietitian or nutritionist. You can search for a practitioner on the British Dietetics Association's Sport and Exercise Nutrition Register (SENR). This is a voluntary register designed to accredit suitably qualified and experienced registrants who have the competency to work autonomously as a sport and exercise nutritionist with performance-oriented athletes, as well as those participating in physical activity, sport and exercise for health. Outside of sport, all dietitians are regulated by the Health & Care Professions Council (HCPC) who publish a register of dietitians and other health professionals who meet their standards. This could be a useful place to search for a dietitian if you or your client are interested in supplements to aid sleep (see the resources section at the end of this book for website details).

SLEEP STRATEGY 6: PHYSICAL ACTIVITY

A major non-pharmacological aid to sleep is physical activity, and it can form an integral part of a person's strategy to get good sleep. Certainly, for women experiencing poor sleep because of, for example, menstrual cycle issues, pregnancy or the menopause transition, regular, safe physical activity can help with sleep in otherwise challenging circumstances.

The terms *physical activity*, *sport*, *exercise* and *physical fitness* often lead to confusion. Originally, I referred to this section of this book as 'sleep strategies and exercise', but to me the term *exercise* is misleading in relation to the benefits for sleep. Really what I mean is physical activity.

Physical activity is any form of movement that results in energy expenditure and includes all activities in day-to-day living, whether professional, domestic or leisure-time activities (Chennaoui *et al.*, 2015). This encompasses all aspects of movement that can help sleep, whether it be a gentle walk around the block, completing a Couch to 5K programme, a Pilates class or training for a marathon.

I also find when advising people about sleep that if I suggest exercise as a strategy to help sleep, then this is sometimes seen as a negative activity. Not everyone loves to exercise. Whereas if I use the term 'physical activity', then people are more likely to engage in this as a useful non-pharmacological intervention to aid sleep. For brevity and standardization, I will refer to sleep and its relationship with physical activity throughout this chapter.

Given physical activity can be complex, causing a stress on the body, it can be hard to relate to how it can aid sleep (Driver & Taylor, 2000), and yet it is widely regarded as a useful facilitator of sleep. It increases heart rate and elevates core body temperature and breathing rate, and certain hormones are released in response to the 'activity stress' – for example, adrenaline and cortisol. Physical activity can also cause dehydration, resulting in restless sleep as one can feel hot, thirsty and uncomfortable during the night. It can also induce muscle soreness which can be painful, last for a few days and upset sleep. When you look at physical activity at face value, it seems hard to justify how it can be seen as a sleep aid, and yet it is a strong source of tiredness and the onset of sleep.

As you might expect, when it comes to sleep and physical activity, the relationship is reciprocal, complex and intricate, involving multiple physiological and psychological pathways (Chennaoui, et al., 2016; Thun et al., 2015; Banno et al., 2018; Bjornsdottir, 2024). The complexity of the relationship can make giving recommendations around sleep and physical activity difficult, but the fundamental point is that any form of physical activity will aid sleep. Conversely, if a person sleeps poorly, they are less motivated to engage in some form of physical activity. Therefore, suboptimal sleep may contribute to low physical activity levels and this has obvious ramifications for long-term health (Kline, 2014).

The many benefits of physical activity for overall health and wellbeing are well documented, not least for improving the health of countless people with chronic diseases, such as obesity, type 2 diabetes and cardiovascular disease (Chennaoui et al., 2015). Physical activity is also particularly good for women in midlife when, for example, osteoporosis becomes more of a risk factor (Brooke-Wavell et al., 2022). Furthermore, physical activity can often be performed outdoors, helping with the body's exposure to natural light, which is so fundamental to the circadian rhythm and the light–dark cycle that we learnt about in Chapter 2 (Wirz-Justice et al., 2021).

Without a doubt, a person's sleep will benefit hugely from completing some form of physical activity. Typically, people who perform physical activity regularly fall asleep quicker (faster sleep onset latency) and achieve good sleep quality through more stage 3 sleep (deep sleep) and longer sleep (Driver & Taylor, 2000; Kredlow *et al.*, 2015; Goldberg *et al.*, 2024). This is good news since deep sleep solidifies new memories, reduces anxiety, stimulates the immune system, regulates appetite, lowers blood sugar and regulates blood pressure (Halson, 2014).

Suboptimal sleep also has an impact on cognitive abilities and sport performance. Cognitive factors typically affected by poor sleep are executive function,[7] attention, learning and mental performance. Performance parameters affected by suboptimal sleep tend to be strength, coordination, speed and endurance, with greater effects seen on tasks requiring precision (Mellow *et al.*, 2022). Linked to this, reaction time, decision making and memory may also be affected, all critical to many forms of physical activity.

Except for fast, explosive anaerobic events such as sprinting, where the impact of sleep loss is marginal, numerous recreational activities are affected by restricted sleep (Reilly & Edwards, 2007; Halson, 2008). It is often the psycho-physiological perspective that can influence sports performance when sleep is restricted. Participants in low-aerobic, high-vigilance sports such as sailing and road cycling may incur more errors because of sleep restriction. Similarly, concentration is affected in moderate aerobic, high-focus sports such as field sports and team games. In sports where there is a mix of aerobic and anaerobic demands, such as combat sports or middle-distance events, there seems to be a loss of power from sleep restriction (Reilly & Edwards, 2007; Halson, 2008). So, a variety of sports are affected by poor sleep.

Unsurprisingly, the transfer of chronic suboptimal sleep to the field of play may also increase the risk of exercise-induced injury (Chennaoui *et al.*, 2015; Huang & Ihm, 2021). The amount of sleep that consistently has been found to be associated with increased risk of exercise-induced injury is less than seven hours of sleep, which, when sustained for periods of at least 14 days, has been associated with 1.7 times greater risk of musculoskeletal injury (Huang & Ihm, 2021). However, it is not clear whether improved sleep translates to reduced incidence of sport-related injury. Injury risk is multifaceted, with sleep being just one of the parameters that is associated with it. Further, studies focusing on musculoskeletal injury risk and sleep have tended to use subjective measures of sleep, with

---

7   Executive function is an umbrella term for a wide range of higher-order cognitive processes that coordinate a person's skills needed for planning, initiation and control of complex, independent, appropriate and purposeful goal-directed behaviour (Reimers, 2019).

limited objective measures of sleep and injury risk being available (Burke *et al.*, 2020). Nevertheless, it is possible that sleep interventions have a positive impact on the prevention of musculoskeletal injuries (Grier *et al.*, 2020). So, if your client is engaging in a new skill in the gym, or aiming to increase their training load, especially when in a transition phase such as moving from the offseason to a training camp (Huang & Ihm, 2021), perhaps first ensure that they are getting enough sleep.

The focus on injury risk and sleep is particularly important for women when you consider the recent rise in focus on female health matters, sport and injury risk (Moore *et al.*, 2023). Certainly, the increased media attention on women's sport in recent years has brought into the spotlight the inequality of support for, and lack of understanding of, the health and physiological needs of women and girls across sport (UK Parliament, 2024). Thankfully, lots of work is being done in the science and medicine spheres to rectify this, so keep an eye on research outlets for updates.

The link between physical activity and sleep can be influenced by several factors, such as individual characteristics (e.g. age, gender, fitness level, type of sleeper, body mass index (BMI)) and exercise regime and protocol. The latter includes the type (aerobic or anaerobic; cardiovascular or resistance), frequency (acute or chronic), intensity (endurance or high intensity), duration, environment and timing of exercise (Driver & Taylor, 2000; Chennaoui *et al.*, 2015; Thun *et al.*, 2015). Each of these factors may have an influence on sleep, although the effects are subtle. For example, changes in rapid eye movement (REM) sleep is considered a sensitive marker of the exercise effects on sleep. Exercise is significantly correlated with the decrease of REM sleep as more deep sleep (slow-wave NREM sleep) is observed (Wang & Boros, 2021). Regardless, these effects are subtle, and it is much better, for sleep and overall health, for a person to be performing some form of physical activity, rather than nothing at all in fear of disrupting their sleep architecture.

Regarding the exercise regime and protocol, let us look at *timing* first as I get asked the 'When is the best time to perform physical activity?' question a lot in my sleep education sessions. The answer is it is individualized, like all aspects of sleep, but ideally a person should do some form of physical activity when they can reasonably fit it into their schedule, without compromising too much on other areas such as good nutrition and a regular sleep routine. Modern-day living means people are often time-poor, and fitting in physical activity can be a challenge.

Commonly, for those with busy family, social and work commitments, physical activity is either squeezed into an early morning or evening session. Whilst this isn't an issue generally, it can have a subsequent effect on sleep quality and quantity if not managed correctly.

Regarding late-night exercise, historically, advice has been to limit this due to the effect is has on an individual in terms of levels of alertness, hunger and an increased core body temperature following exercise (humans need to be cool to aid sleep onset). However, more recent studies have reported that exercise in the evening makes little difference to sleep provided it is managed well (Stutz, Eiholzer & Spengler, 2019; Miller et al., 2020). Generally speaking, if an individual exercises in the evening, they should ideally aim to have finished more than an hour before bedtime with optimal recovery – for example, stretch, have a warm bath and a recovery snack. It's highly unlikely that they would finish exercise and immediately get into bed! Good-quality sleep is the focus in this scenario, so if exercise finishes late in the evening, advise your clients to have bedtime a little later that night so they are ready for sleep onset, and sacrifice the quantity of sleep, so they get slightly less, but good-quality sleep. The following night, they should aim to resume a normal bedtime schedule and routine.

Physical activity across different times of the day will aid sleep health (Goldberg et al., 2024). Whilst there are subtle differences in sleep architecture with activity at different times of the day, these differences are minimal, and the main theme is that an individual will get plenty of sleep benefits whatever time of day they perform some physical activity. Physical activity, independent of the time at which it takes place, leads to extended NREM sleep without other effects on sleep quality (Goldberg et al., 2024). Therefore, it has been advised that, considering the crucial role of physical activity in achieving good wellbeing, sleep health guidelines should promote it at any time of the day (Goldberg et al., 2024).

For frequency and intensity of physical activity relating to sleep, the advice is similar to general physical activity guidelines. The American College of Sports Medicine and the American Heart Association promotes moderate-intensity aerobic exercise for 30 minutes for five days a week, or vigorous-intensity aerobic physical activity for 20 minutes over three days a week, as being beneficial to health (Chennaoui et al., 2015). This happily parallels the advice around frequency and intensity of physical activity for aiding sleep, where 30 minutes of moderate exercise three times a week is typically suggested to see a positive change in a person's sleep, particularly for older people (Vanderlinden, Boen & van Uffelen, 2020).

As for type of physical activity and sleep, there may be subtle differences in sleep architecture using one form of exercise versus another, such as aerobic or resistance exercise, but overall, both types of physical activity benefit sleep (Gupta, Bansal & Saxena, 2022)

In terms of the timing, frequency, duration and intensity of physical activity, it makes little difference in terms of the benefits to sleep health how long, to what intensity and how many times an individual performs an exercise bout. For intensity of exercise, whilst vigorous exercise can have a positive effect on sleep, especially in younger people, moderate exercise has displayed more promising outcomes on sleep quality. However, in some cases, vigorous exercise pre-sleep has had a negative effect on sleep (Oda & Shirakawa, 2014). Therefore, the intensity of activity needs to be taken into consideration when researching the relationship between physical activity and sleep quality (Wang & Boros, 2021). To aid sleep, any movement, at any time of day, is better than being sedentary (Goldberg *et al.*, 2024). Fitting physical activity into a day is often hard with the demands of work, family life and socializing, so finding an activity that successfully helps an individual move regularly is advised.

The positive effect on sleep is not dose dependent either: a person doesn't have to perform more physical activity over time to reap the same sleep benefits. The consistency of physical activity over time is fundamental to aiding sleep, however, in that the positive association between sleep and physical activity is lost if a person is initially active, but then becomes inactive (Bjornsdottir *et al.*, 2024).

Relatively sedate forms of physical activity can also help with relaxation before sleep. Mind–body exercise, such as yoga or tai-chi, has been shown to have a positive effect on sleep and mood, adding to the management of not only sleep but also mental health issues (Siddarth, Siddarth & Lavretsky, 2014). Such exercise modalities maybe a good tactic to help a person unwind before bed, if they enjoy this type of exercise.

Another important consideration with sleep and physical activity is the interaction of age. As a person grows older, it can become harder to generate deep sleep. Studies investigating elderly populations and physical activity have found the cognitive function of older people is sharper after exercise-enhanced deep sleep and that exercise programmes positively affect various aspects of sleep (Vanderlinden *et al.*, 2020).

Whilst moderate exercise has been shown to have positive effects on sleep in older people, for younger people the suggestion seems to be that the exercise intensity needs to be more vigorous to have any positive effect on sleep. Studies on physical activity and sleep in younger populations have yielded mixed results, with different methodologies making conclusions hard to draw. However, often for younger people in research studies, light or moderate exercise didn't yield the same sizeable enhancement of deep sleep compared to older populations, whereas vigorous exercise did (Dolezal *et al.*, 2017; Fonseca *et al.*, 2021). Adolescents, therefore, generally must perform more vigorous exercise to see the sleep improvements seen in their older counterparts. Also, in adolescents, higher levels of physical fitness were associated with longer nocturnal sleep periods and better sleep quality.

Sleep in adolescence is a particular challenge. Teenagers have a greater sleep need than adults, but less than in childhood. There is also a conflict between the biological delay of sleep times in adolescents (the circadian rhythm shift) and social factors, such as morning school schedules (a strong synchronizer of wake-up time over a week) (Dolezal *et al.*, 2017; Fonseca *et al.*, 2021). Sometimes in this demographic, exercise can affect the opportunity to get good sleep. In other words, with younger people, the time needed to complete physical activity can sometimes hinder their social time, if it is not the same activity. This then compromises the sleep window, and adolescents therefore try to cram all aspects of their lives – for example, schooling, exercise, study and socializing – into too short a wake window.

In summary, in answer to the question of whether physical activity is good for sleep, the answer is yes! On the whole, the research suggests that physical activity can improve sleep quality without notable adverse effects. Beneficial effects of regular physical activity on sleep may be explained in a multitude of ways, with the interaction of circadian rhythm, metabolic, immune, thermoregulatory, vascular, mood and endocrine effects. However, to reach a full agreement on whether sleep and physical activity exert significant positive effects on one another, the mechanisms behind these observations need to be verified (Banno *et al.*, 2018). Differences in the exercise protocols studied (e.g. aerobic or anaerobic, intensity and duration) and interactions between individual characteristics (e.g. fitness, age and gender) cloud the current experimental evidence supporting a sleep-enhancing effect of physical activity. Further, studies have often included good, relatively young sleepers and not focused on older subjects. Equally, studies have sometimes assessed exercise and sleep using instruments of dubious validity or tended to not include clinical diagnoses of sleep disorders (Youngstedt & Kline, 2006). New fundamental research must be carried out to improve our knowledge of the complex physiological effects and to understand the benefit of exercise for sleep health in both healthy subjects and patients (Driver & Taylor, 2000; Thun *et al.*, 2015; Dolezal *et al.*, 2017; Wang & Boros, 2021; Alnawwar *et al.*, 2023). More age-group-specific research is also needed to develop detailed exercise suggestions in order to make accurate recommendations for health promotion in relation to sleep (Vanderlinden *et al.*, 2020; Wang & Boros, 2021).

Nevertheless, the positive generic effects of physical activity on sleep cannot be overlooked. Physical activity is recommended as an alternative or complementary approach to existing therapies for sleep problems and can be advocated as an effective non-pharmacological intervention for sleep disorders or conditions leading to disordered sleeping, such as cardiovascular disease, type 2 diabetes, depression and some cancers (Yang *et al.*, 2012; Dolezal *et al.*, 2017; Banno *et al.*, 2018; Wang & Boros, 2021). But remember that the implementation of physical activity needs to consider participants' age and health status (Wang & Boros, 2021).

The bottom line is moving is good for sleep, but ensure clients *enjoy* rather than *endure* the physical activity bout (Wang & Boros, 2021). Advise clients to find something that works for them and regularly commit to it throughout their week. Recognize that fitting physical activity into a day is often hard with the demands of work, family life and socializing, and remind them to be wary of timing and whether it seems to affect their ability to obtain optimal sleep. If not, then continue with their physical activity programme, but if sleep is affected by the timing of their activity, where possible modify this to accommodate for getting good sleep. Always ensure a client is physically safe and able to perform their chosen physical activity and regularly encourage its use for aiding good sleep.

SLEEP STRATEGY 7: SLEEP AIDS

Sleep aids are typically gadgets or accessories brought to market with the promise of aiding sleep. Sleep aids fall under the umbrella of 'strategies for sleep' as they can sometimes help in a person's quest for sleep onset. What follows are some pointers based on some of the most common questions that I am asked in relation to sleep aids. The list is by no means exhaustive; other options to help improve sleep health are available and sleep health innovations come to market frequently, but I hope this information enables you to have an informed dialogue about which sleep aid might be a good option for your client to help improve their sleep health. As ever, practical strategies should be employed first (e.g. a good sleep routine), not least because they are often free or inexpensive, compared to the multitude of, often expensive, sleep aids available, all purporting to improve sleep.

Technological

In addition to the laboratory methods and clinical field measures to measure sleep mentioned in Chapter 2, contemporary technologies for sleep assessment (namely sleep trackers) have exploded onto the consumer marketplace in recent years (Byrne, 2017). This is thanks mostly to the boost in the wellness industry, which is worth billions of dollars, and sleep tracker technologies are an integral part of it.

Sleep trackers are an ever-changing sleep aid, with a wealth of gadgets and applications claiming to monitor and improve sleep (Saner, 2019). These are often referred to as 'wearable and nearable technologies' (sometimes unbearable!) and include examples such as smartphone applications, smart watches and bedside sleep devices.

On the one hand, sleep tracker technology has encouraged an increased awareness of sleep and its invaluable role in supporting optimal physical and mental health. Good news for improving global sleep health. On the other hand, such wearables can be guilty of promoting sleep as an issue to be addressed, rather than as an area of natural human function which can be illustrated on an individual level through wearable technology (Saner, 2019). Whilst some people may need help in improving their sleep health, others may have good sleep and not need to place an unnecessary objective focus on it. Sometimes gleaning objective feedback from an individual's sleep bout can potentially create a concomitant reliance on the sleep technologies informing them if they have slept well or not.

From this potential reliance, an emerging trend in relation to the downside of sleep trackers is 'orthosomnia'. Coming from the word 'ortho', meaning 'correct' or 'perfect', it is likened to the term 'orthorexia' where patients have a damaging obsession with eating healthily. Orthosomnia is not a formal sleep disorder, but it describes a tendency to place undue importance on the data from personal sleep tracking devices. Some readers may have seen a client who has an obsessive pursuit of optimal sleep that is driven by their sleep tracker data and are experiencing poor sleep because of overthinking this objective data.

Personality type certainly plays a part in orthosomnia. If a client has issues with their sleep or is the type of person who would be anxious if their sleep is suboptimal, objectively tracking how much sleep they are getting and its quality can become an unhealthy fixation. Although not a specific sleep disorder itself, orthosomnia can be present alongside other sleep disorders, such as insomnia. It can potentially exacerbate sleep problems and may persist even after a primary sleep disorder has been successfully treated (Summer & Rehman, 2022).

My advice in these instances is to tell your client to put their sleep tracker in another room when they go to bed and speak to a psychologist with regard to an intervention to aid sleep, such as cognitive behavioural therapy for insomnia.

An interest in sleep and a casual glance at some objective data gathered over time, when trying to make a change to a sleep routine, may be helpful, but obsessively poring over a single night's sleep tracker data is not a healthy habit and, in terms of the data, not actually that meaningful.

Whilst there is a place for sleep technologies in monitoring a change in a person's sleep pattern, unfortunately, not all contemporary sleep measurement technologies measure accurately what they claim to. Part of the problem is that the billion-dollar sleep technology industry is moving at a fast pace and products are coming to the market sooner than regulators or scientists can review them. The danger is that sleep trackers become a purely commercial product with the scientific surveillance required for their quality assurance ignored (Purtill, 2024). Multiple validation studies have demonstrated consumer-wearable sleep-tracking devices are unable to precisely discriminate stages of sleep and have poor accuracy in detecting wake after sleep onset (Baron *et al.*, 2017). As we learnt in Chapter 2, the gold standard measure of sleep quality and quantity is polysomnography (PSG), the laboratory-based method of assessing brain waves during sleep. Whilst wearable and nearable sleep measurement technologies are a cheaper alternative to such scientifically validated equipment, and more user-friendly in the field, they can be counterproductive to good sleep.

Although sleep technologies are frequently reported to help assess sleep, frequently they are absent from any form of quality assurance as to the data produced and how consistent they are. Often they take some aspects of medical-grade methodologies but fail to validate them against the gold-standard quality assurance measure of sleep (PSG). Consequently, they fail to provide an accurate assessment of an individual's sleep characteristics and quality. Some next-generation sleep wearables or nearables purport to measure sleep stages (NREM and REM sleep), yet this is an indirect measure of sleep, as it is most likely attached to a wrist, hand or even under a pillow, and therefore, at best, can only infer sleep from a physiological measure, such as heart rate or breathing rate, compared to the gold standard brain wave technologies observing actual sleep architecture, as with PSG (Byrne, 2017).

However, to the person experiencing orthosomnia, sleep tracker data often feels more consistent with their experience of sleep than validated techniques, such as polysomnography or actigraphy. The challenge for practitioners is balancing educating clients on the validity of sleep technology devices with patients' enthusiasm for objective data (Baron *et al.*, 2017).

More recent high-quality sleep trackers available on the market do seem to produce reasonable results for some sleep markers, such as sleep efficiency (Ong *et al.*, 2024). But where an individual has poor sleep efficiency, sleep trackers may not be the best tool to assess their sleep. However, what they will be useful for is as a tool for monitoring changes. So if an individual is using some practical strategies to make a positive alteration to their sleep health, then a sleep wearable will help them quantify that change. What it won't do is inform them of a clinical sleep issue or provide accurate information about the architecture of their sleep quality and quantity. For that they need a sleep laboratory.

Technology provides an enormous opportunity for general health monitoring, not least sleep monitoring. Aside from sleep trackers measuring solely sleep data, over the last few years numerous methods and techniques have been developed to record other vital body parameters such as respiratory and cardiac activity from within or around the bed (Van Deun *et al.*, 2015). A lot of these advances in sleep technology have been possible through the development of artificial intelligence, meaning some sleep technologies can now aid sleep health through informing the user how the body is responding during the night and how to make changes accordingly. For example, with regard to body temperature, high heat capacity mattresses, compared to conventional low heat capacity mattresses, can increase conductive body heat loss which enhances the nocturnal decline in core body temperature. This may then be accompanied by an increase in slow-wave sleep, and therefore increased subjective sleep quality and sleep stability (Kräuchi *et al.*, 2018).

The manipulation of body temperature during sleep may be a useful approach to enhance sleep in postmenopausal women and could potentially also have a positive impact on the sleep system options for perimenopausal women experiencing vasomotor symptoms that cause nighttime wakenings (Reid *et al.*, 2021). In terms of future innovations, the bedroom holds an enormous opportunity for artificial intelligence applications that can do exactly what is needed: assist the user in a sensible manner, learn their preferences and react to their frame of mind and needs (Van Deun *et al.*, 2015). For sleep technologies looking to assist a person's sleep quality and quantity, this could be an absolute game changer.

In summary, if you are going to advise about investing in a technology to help measure sleep, remember that the absolute data may not be as accurate as hoped. In the absence of a sleep laboratory, a good method for a person to assess their sleep quality and quantity is to subjectively assess how they feel upon waking and if they are alert, refreshed and fully productive during the working day.

Light therapy

Light therapy, or phototherapy, is an intervention to help certain sleep disorders through exposure to light of a particular illuminance (brightness, measured in lux). Light therapy works by imitating outdoor light and delivering it through a light box or, more directly, through light glasses. Glasses offer a suitable alternative to a light box due to the length of exposure required to reap the benefits of light therapy (typically 30–60 minutes). Owing to the proximity of the light glasses to the eye, the intensity of light used will be slightly less than when using a light box.

Light therapy is most effective when there is the proper combination of light intensity, duration and timing, which ultimately are dependent on the disorder being treated, but usually first thing in the morning is best, with consistent use until symptoms subside.

Benefits of light therapy may generally include improved sleepiness, enhanced vigilance and cognition, improved mood and consequently a reduced risk of accidents (Comtet *et al.*, 2019). To be safe and assured that a person has the correct protocol for effective treatment – that is, brightness (intensity), timing, duration and type of light – they should have a dialogue with their GP before attempting light therapy. It also goes without saying that clients should be advised to always follow medical recommendations and manufacturers' guidelines.

Weighted blankets

Weighted blankets have been shown to decrease anxiety and potentially improve sleep quality and quantity. They are a form of deep pressure therapy, a technique used widely for people with autism spectrum disorders, anxiety and some other disorders and disabilities (Bestbier & Williams, 2017).

Deep pressure therapy works on the theory that the whole body can respond to firm contact such as hugging, squeezing or compression in a way that can help lower physiological arousal (stress) through reducing the autonomic nervous system's normal responses to stress (i.e. excitatory).[8]

Weighted blankets contain small plastic pellets and ball bearings that make them feel much heavier than a standard duvet. This helps the feeling of touch and the associated relaxation it can bring. Different weights are available, but generally it is suggested to sleep with a blanket that is 10 per cent of an individual's body weight. However, how comfortable a person may feel is entirely subjective, so trial and error may be required. Take note that purchasing several different weighted blankets could become expensive.

Importantly, ensure the weighted blanket is breathable. Adding an extra blanket may make a person too warm and having the right temperature environment to sleep in (usually around 18–20°C) is critical in helping a person to fall and stay asleep.

There is a huge variety of weighted blankets on the market, including lighter ones for children. Always speak to a GP before using a weighted blanket for a child, and note that they are not advised for children under three to four years of age. For adults, many types of weighted blanket are marketed, but I often advise people to try using a folded blanket from home first and see if that makes a difference to their sleep, as this can be a more cost-effective alternative.

Because the concept of a weighted blanket for sleep health is

---

8   The autonomic nervous system regulates involuntary physiologic processes including heart rate, blood pressure, respiration, digestion and sexual arousal (Waxenbaum, Reddy & Varacallo, 2023).

relatively new and the benefits are not well known, more research is needed as to the exact mechanisms and benefits of using weighted blankets to help improve sleep.

Eye masks and ear plugs

Noise and light are certainly annoying if a person is experiencing difficulties in falling or staying asleep. It is widely known that eye masks and ear plugs can be a useful and simple strategy in limiting these irritations before sleep and promoting good sleep health overall.

Whilst blue light may not have the negative effects on sleep previously thought, bright lights remain a problem in delaying sleep onset. Where there is unavoidable light in the bedroom, such as from streetlights, try suggesting clients use not only eye masks but also blackout blinds or curtains. Minimizing light exposure before bed allows melatonin levels to rise, which then causes the feelings of sleepiness and aids sleep onset.

There are many types of ear plugs available, from traditional foam ear plugs to wax or silicon. The technology around ear plugs is quite sophisticated nowadays, with white-noise-emitting ear plugs and ear plugs that block out different sound frequencies being available. At the end of the day, it comes down to cost, comfort and personal preference. The optimal type of ear plug is one that stays in, is comfortable throughout the night and blocks out noise.

Whilst various types of masks and ear plugs exist on the market, the key is finding ones that are comfortable for the individual and don't interfere with their sleep, be it the time taken to fall asleep (sleep onset latency) or sleep quantity or quality through causing nighttime waking.

SLEEP STRATEGY 8: RELAXATION TECHNIQUES

Relaxation techniques can be useful to help create the best environment pre-sleep and there are a whole host of calming activities that can aid sleep. It may be mindfulness, breathing exercises, mind–body exercise such as yoga, listening to music or reading that have the desired effect; it really is up to the individual how they relax.

Some techniques may require a more specialized intervention – for example, cognitive behavioural therapy for insomnia (CBT-I) or another psychological technique, acceptance and commitment therapy

(ACT).[9] Both methods have been shown to help with ongoing sleep problems and are a good alternative to medication, but you should advise people to seek medical guidance for these support mechanisms. Chapter 7 covered CBT-1 in more detail, along with the digital technologies for CBT-1 that are increasingly available to aid sleep.

Other more accessible techniques can be performed independently in the home. Specific guidelines for relaxation activities can be researched individually depending on what motivates a person. For pre-sleep relaxation, it is very much an individualized approach, with people adhering to different methods for success. Sometimes simple relaxation techniques such as reading or listening to music may be all that is needed. Other times it may be that commitment to a specific activity (such as CBT-1) is required for a successful sleep health outcome. Where sleep frequently eludes your clients, either through problems getting to sleep or frequent night wakings, seek medical advice.

If travelling, sleep is often disturbed due to an inability to relax and unfamiliarity with the new environment, and is rarely preventable. This 'first night effect' means an individual may have a relatively poor night's sleep the first night in their new sleep surroundings as they familiarize. However, this decreases the longer they are in the new environment. Sleep disturbances can also be minimized by making the room they sleep in feel like home, so advise people to bring small items of bedding, such as a pillow, to help with relaxation and the familiarity of the environment for sleep.

If an individual is away with work and has work to do in the evening, working outside of their hotel room, such as in the hotel lounge, and only going to the bedroom when ready to sleep is helpful. Ideally, the body should associate the bedroom and bedtime with sleep and not a place for being awake and working. The pre-sleep focus should be on disarming any pre-sleep arousals and being relaxed enough to fall asleep.

New generation technologies arise frequently, for example, relaxation rhythms in the form of audio frequencies mimicking brain waves during sleep, so always ensure you advise a client to follow GP and manufacturers' recommendations if using new sleep aid technologies.

---

9   Acceptance and commitment therapy (ACT) is a form of talking therapy that emphasizes acceptance to deal with negative thoughts, feelings, symptoms or circumstances. It encourages increased commitment to healthy, constructive activities that uphold a person's values or goals.

SLEEP STRATEGY 9: MEDICATIONS

Medications for aiding sleep fall outside the scope of my technical knowledge as I am not a medical doctor, but it is important to mention them in a chapter about sleep aids.

Clearly, sleep medications have undergone rigorous clinical trials to test their efficacy and safety for use on the general public; however, they are not a quick or easy fix for sleep problems.

If your client is struggling with their sleep and doesn't have a sleep or circadian rhythm disorder, then they should aim to try some of the non-pharmacological, practical strategies outlined in this chapter to help their sleep before considering prescription medication. And if a client is suffering from the sleep disorder insomnia, then CBT-I is seen as the primary first-line treatment. Similarly, if a client suffers from sleep-disordered breathing, then clinical interventions such as CPAP maybe appropriate over pharmacological solutions.

If medication is required to help a client's sleep, then it should be with a full consultation with their GP and only used as a short-term solution. The situation should then be monitored and reviewed regularly with a clear plan to cease taking the medication at an appropriate time. Unfortunately, this is not always the case.

A variety of practical strategies for helping good sleep health have been presented in this chapter. The sleep environment, sleep systems, nutrition, physical activity, sleep aids and relaxation techniques may all potentially help a person achieve good sleep health. In the absence of a sleep disorder, putting in place a sleep strategy with some practical solutions may be all a person needs to avoid poor sleep issues. Where a sleep disorder is suspected, then clinical input is required through the person's GP or through the resources listed at the end of this book.

In attempting to improve sleep quality and quantity, remember that sleep is an entirely individualized process. What works for one person to improve sleep may not work for someone else. Also, how a person copes and responds to poor sleep is individualized and may change throughout their lifetime. It's important to try the suggested techniques in this chapter if a person is experiencing poor sleep, but to attempt one idea at a time; otherwise, knowing and understanding what works for them is difficult. Do recommend, however, that a client doesn't persevere with an aspect of the suggested sleep strategies if it's keeping them awake and causing more stress and ultimately poorer sleep.

Regardless of what sleep aid your client is interested in trying, ensure that they have the basics in place first – a consistent sleep routine, a good sleep system – and have identified, where possible, anything causing difficulties in getting to sleep or night wakenings. Also, whatever sleep aids your clients are considering, ensure they have sought medical advice, referred to the manufacturer recommendations (where relevant) and have made an evidence-based, informed decision.

The secret weapon of sleep for delivering more effectively at work and in life is free and accessible to all. Without sounding too harsh, the responsibility really is on the individual if they are armed with sleep education and information for support. If they value sleep as something crucial to their life, and take it seriously, then they are in a better position than being ignorant to the fact that sleep is crucial to health. Where possible, prioritizing sleep, personalizing it and protecting it by finding the 'sleep window' will all aid good sleep. In addition, avoiding or preventing things that can upset sleep and trusting that sleep is a natural process will all help an individual to improve their sleep (Espie, 2022a).

CHAPTER 10

Comments on Contemporary Sleep and Closing Remarks

Various contemporary factors need to be considered in relation to sleep, not least the impact of industrialized society on human sleep. Technological advances, along with the habits and behaviours of new generations, mean the human relationship with sleep needs reprioritizing.

Part of this reprioritization of sleep involves educating and advising people about their sleep health. I hope that this book has to some degree enabled you as a practitioner to be able to do just that. Whilst the focus has been on the life cycle of women's sleep, some of the narrative is transferable to sleep in society as a whole.

This chapter focuses on some of the contemporary factors relating to sleep, sociological discussions around sleep, methods for training sleep practitioners and future directions in the field of sleep health, not just for women's health, but for wider society too.

SOCIETY AND SLEEP

Industrialized society can be against improving sleep health. Where light can be described as the sleep robber, industrialization and consumerism can be similarly labelled as the enemies of sleep. In an age where cities are famous for never sleeping, some shops are open 24 hours a day, seven days a week, plus, of course, the revolution in technology and the innovation of the internet, humans can live in a world that never switches off and consumers can access anything they want, at any time of day. Unfortunately, all this perpetuates the problem of sleep restriction. Add into the mix the fast pace of life and the 'on demand' culture of younger generations, and sleep is immediately compromised and at odds with contemporary ways of living (Jein, 2020).

How different are current generations' sleep from that of their ancestors? Certainly, cultural shifts, migration and technological advancements are considered factors in the evolution of sleep. Before the Middle Ages, sleep was a communal affair, most likely for warmth and safety (Walker, 2024c). Theories around sleep in the Middle Ages onwards suggest humans had a biphasic[1] sleep pattern involving a first sleep from approximately nine or ten o'clock in the evening until approximately one o'clock in the morning, with a further sleep from around three o'clock in the morning until sunrise. The probable reason for this two-phase sleep was to keep people aware of the dangers of predators and allow chores to be completed. Later evidence suggests that generally people used the time to converse, or if sleeping in private rooms, for physical intimacy (Gorvett, 2022).

Segmented sleep continued and civilization remained in the dark once the sun set for many years. The infamous 18th-century informal learned society of Lunar Men[2] were so named as they would only hold their dynamic, intellectual meetings if there was a full moon, as the extra light made the journey home easier and safer in the absence of street lighting. Imagine how many more theories, philosophies and social reforms would have been discussed had street lighting been invented in the 1700s!

Biphasic sleep disappeared from society once the 19th-century industrial revolution occurred, and from the 1800s to the present day, sleep has evolved to being a much more consolidated single bout of nighttime sleep (monophasic sleep). Though it seems, unfortunately, that this sleep block is becoming shorter generation by generation.

As civilization developed and became more industrialized, society in general became louder and lighter at night with, for example, the invention of the lightbulb, and thus streetlights. Added to this was the fact that people generally worked a more regimented nine-to-five working day. This meant sleeping in segments and napping whenever required became

---

1   Biphasic sleep describes a pattern of sleep in which a person sleeps in two segments, or phases, per day as opposed to monophasic sleep, which is a single bout of sleep, typically nocturnal.

2   A meeting of friends who gathered in the Birmingham, UK, area for lively dinner conversations, led by the intellectual Erasmus Darwin. The group included famous innovators, philosophers and entrepreneurs such as James Watt, Joseph Priestley and Josiah Wedgwood.

less practical and a longer monophasic nocturnal sleep period became the norm. Fast-forward to current times, and the contemporary world is not geared up for long, calm sleep bouts. Thanks to the surge in manufacturing, industry and technological innovations, humans no longer have little to do in the late evening and sleep-restricting activities abound. In modern society, people can access everything at their fingertips, whenever they want, 24 hours a day. For example, rolling news cycles, binge-watching the latest television series and social media all impact on a person's opportunity to sleep at night.

In addition, some working practices no longer have boundaries or are regimented as traditional nine-to-five hours, so often intrude into the evenings. Fryer (2006) reported that in today's society the need to work long hours (e.g. 100-plus-hour work weeks) and frequent crossing of multiple time zones are the kinds of corporate behaviour that are the antithesis of high performance. These behaviours, plus other lifestyle factors related to a modern 24/7 society, such as psychosocial stress, unbalanced diet, lack of physical activity and excessive electronic media use, actually worsen productivity in the workplace, provoke poor sleep and cause physical and mental health problems both short and long term. This is not great for thriving in the workplace or in society, and I elaborate on the impact of poor sleep on industry later in this chapter.

Further, sleep, or more broadly rest, is political. The people who have little opportunity in society, whether that be through education, resource or privilege, often work the longest and hardest and rest the least (Mycroft, 2023). Consider the shift worker whose occupation is to clean at night and has other employment during the daytime. This is where the cost of living can have a fundamental impact on a person's ability to regularly sleep well. Socioeconomic factors certainly play a role in sleep education, awareness and opportunity to get good sleep quality and quantity. Indeed, Papadopoulos and Etindele Sosso (2023) reported that socioeconomic deprivation is associated with poorer sleep efficiency, higher frequency of sleep complaints and daytime sleepiness, and lower overall sleep satisfaction.

Equally, one cannot penalize someone if they sleep poorly as sometimes it is due to factors outside of their control. What is helpful is to promote the benefits of being aware of sleep and good strategies to get to sleep. In society, or the workplace even, we rarely celebrate good role models to promote sleep health. Perhaps what is needed are 'sleep role models' in society. In my previous career in high-performance sport, we used role models all the time to display optimal behaviours and create a culture of professionalism around the athletes. For example, those athletes who focused on protecting, prioritizing and valuing their sleep were highlighted in terms of their approach to attempting to give themselves the opportunity to get good sleep quality and quantity on a regular basis. That is not to say those with restricted sleep, or a suspected sleep disorder, weren't supported, but displaying good sleep behaviours was advertised as 'best practice' and even described, in the language of elite sport, as 'gold standard' athlete behaviour. This was relatively easy to do in the more traditional sports, where there was typically a development pathway of talented athletes to elite. Athletes tended to be educated, performance managed in their sport and immersed in a culture where performance-enhancing behaviour such as gaining sufficient sleep was promoted (Bonnar *et al.*, 2019). Athletes received organizational support (athlete and coach education) which was informed by a solid foundation of scientific research, so there was a strong focus on evidence-based science and medicine support practices. Performance-enhancing behaviour was prioritized, which increased the likelihood of competitive success – for example, athletes were more likely to understand the importance of a sleep–wake schedule and avoiding irregular sleep schedules. Training was generally centralized, although it did depend on the sport, and a performance culture was standard and evidence-based behaviour regularly displayed all around the athletes, coaches and support staff (Bonnar *et al.*, 2019).

This performance-enhancing behaviour is much harder to instil in public health, where all levels of society may be struggling with poor sleep. Therefore, perhaps developing good sleep role models in society is one avenue to focus on in terms of education and promoting awareness around sleep in the general public.

MEDIA

Given the reported worldwide decline in sleep quality and quantity, never more so than now have humans needed techniques and strategies to help learn to 'switch off' at bedtime and be self-aware enough to not be on devices beyond their sleep time. However, this is easier said than done, and aside from the culture of sleep in society tending to be to 'just get by on what sleep I get', the mass media sometimes perpetuate unhelpful messages about sleep. Bravado can be reported in the media from individuals claiming to need little sleep; for example, the ex-British prime minister Baroness Margaret Thatcher had notorious indefatigability and helped to exacerbate the myth that the less sleep you need, the more efficient an individual you are. Unfortunately, this is not the case, and it is here the media can be guilty of sensationalizing sleep stories for journalistic gain. Similar comments made by other prominent figures in society about needing a small amount of sleep have also been reported. Thomas Edison, the famous inventor, reportedly only required about three to four hours of sleep each night and regarded sleep as 'a heritage from our cave days', suggesting that sleep was an activity with limited importance in modern industrialized society. Several global industry leaders reportedly manage on minimal sleep. Dame Helena Morrissey, the British financier, has been described as saying she manages between five and six hours sleep a night, gets up at five in the morning (sometimes earlier) and begins work until her children (of which there are nine!) get up. Similarly, Apple's chief executive officer, Tim Cook, apparently wakes up every day at 3:45 a.m. and begins working. In an international survey about the sleep of leaders and professionals, the findings reported a 'generally sleep-deprived population whose primary barriers to sleep have to do with work, and in particular a failure to psychologically detach from it' (Svetieva, Clerkin & Ruderman, 2017). This is an alarming trend for the next generation of leaders; the minimal sleep approach is not a good strategy for long-term health. Sleep is individualized, but minimal sleep is not something a person could maintain over a long period of time without significantly impacting their health.

Reporting these industry leaders as needing relatively small amounts of sleep sometimes gives the impression that compromising on sleep equals success, which is a dangerous association for long-term health. Whilst some people can be healthy with less sleep than guidelines suggest, we know that chronic poor sleep has an association with certain disease states further down an individual's lifespan, such as dementia, which, incidentally, Baroness Margaret Thatcher lived with in later life.

If your clients are happy with their sleep quality and quantity and feel refreshed and productive during the daytime, then you shouldn't need to advise them about getting more sleep. However, if a client isn't getting a lot of sleep and reporting signs and symptoms of sleep restriction (e.g. daytime sleepiness, mood swings and a lack of motivation to do some form of physical activity), you may need to direct them to the practical strategies outlined in Chapter 9 for obtaining good sleep or even signpost them to appropriate medical help.

SLEEP AND INDUSTRY

Whilst a lack of sleep is thought of as an individual issue, the consequences of insufficient sleep can be far-reaching and dramatic, and can have wider societal and economic effects.

In 2016, RAND, a non-profit institution that helps improve policy and decision making through research and analysis, conducted a study on the economic costs of insufficient sleep, involving five OECD (Organization for Economic Co-operation and Development) countries, including the UK. They found poor sleep was costing the UK economy a whopping £40 billion productivity loss and 200,000 lost working days every year due to sleep-related issues. These could be illness related to sleep loss, or health and safety difficulties causing absenteeism (employees not being at work) or presenteeism (employees being at work but working at a suboptimal level). Alarmingly, the estimates are that the cost of sleep loss to the UK economy will rise to £47 billion by 2030 (Hafner *et al.*, 2017).

Not to minimize the UK economy's productivity issues with sleep, the same study also reported that the USA suffers the biggest financial loss due to sleep restriction among its workforce (up to $411 billion) and has the most working days lost (1.2 million). They were closely followed by Japan, with a financial loss of up to $138 billion and around 600,000 working days lost due to sleep-related issues (RAND, 2016). If nothing else, this highlights the global problem of poor sleep. Whilst companies regularly have policies for helping and protecting employees from the dangers of, for example, smoking and poor nutrition, sleep is often ignored in industry despite its performance-enhancing qualities.

It's not just productivity in the workplace that can be affected by poor sleep. Disastrous health and safety consequences have been seen over time, frequently linked to shift workers. This demographic is at a considerable risk of fatigue-related accidents in the workplace if their shift patterns are not managed appropriately.

Chapter 8 discussed shift work, which is common in many safety-critical industries such as healthcare, manufacturing and transport; unfortunately, some of the biggest international disasters have been linked to the poor sleep of shift work employees. For example, in 1986 the USA's Space Shuttle Challenger exploded shortly after take-off, killing all the seven brave astronauts on board. Reportedly, a lack of sleep and sleep-deprived shift work led to poor decisions being made when launching the shuttle (Mitler *et al.*, 1988). Reports stated that vital managers had been working since one in the morning on the day of the explosion, and they had slept less than two hours the previous night. The consequences for those on board the shuttle, their families, those on the ground in the control room and the wider space exploration community were catastrophic.

Similarly tragic and on a more global scale, the 1986 Chernobyl Nuclear Power Plant disaster was attributed to human error due to sleep restriction as the engineers working on the night of the disaster had been on shift for more than 13 hours. Hundreds of people died directly or indirectly from the explosion – according to the World Health Organization, the exact figure may never be known. There remains a 19-mile exclusion radius around the power plant, with the area considered unfit for human life for the next 50,000 years. It is regarded, at the time of writing, as the worst nuclear power plant catastrophe in history.

Nearer home, according to the UK Parliamentary Office of Science and Technology (Houses of Parliament, 2018), employees in the National Health Service[3] are at a higher risk of sleep or circadian disorders from night work, long hours and on-call work. This leads to quite profound concerns over patient safety and a potential increased risk of medical errors associated with working longer hours: a huge red flag to medical governance agencies, and the UK government in general, that they need to recognize poor sleep as not only an industry-specific but also a significant public health issue.

Suggested industry solutions to the problem of sleep loss and work productivity are that employers could recognize the importance of sleep, and their role in its promotion and education. Means of achieving this could be through designing and building brighter workspaces, combating workplace psychosocial risks, such as unrealistic time pressures, and discouraging the extended use of electronic devices. In support of this,

---

3   The National Health Service (NHS) is one of the largest employers of shift workers in the UK, of which women form a substantial proportion.

public health authorities could encourage employers to pay attention to sleep issues and recognize the benefits of educating their employees about sleep health. Certainly, whilst the impact of insufficient sleep represents a major public health concern, which may be best addressed by changes in an individual's behaviour, this can also be supported by employers and public-policy measures (Grandner *et al.*, 2010a). Parallel to this, the Sleep Charity have an excellent 'Workplace Sleep Ambassador' training programme which focuses on the need for employers to consider sleep issues as part of their employees' wellbeing and appropriately train professionals whose responsibility it is to support those with sleep issues.

Individuals could also take more responsibility for their own sleep health and consider the fact that they could be investing in it more to enable them to be more productive in the workplace and feel better for life in general. Reframing thought processes around work productivity to be less about being busy and more about investing in health, in particular sleep, will have a subsequent beneficial effect on daytime productivity and quality of work.

DIFFERENT GENERATIONS AND SLEEP

As mentioned in Chapter 2, Generation Z is the demographic cohort born in the late 1990s through to the early 2010s. At the time of writing, they are society's teenagers to early 30-year-olds. These individuals have been shown to have poorer sleep restriction than the previous generations of Baby Boomers (born 1946–64), Generation X (born 1965–80) and Millennials (born 1981–96). It's probably not too wide an assumption to make that this generation's sleep restriction is, in large part, due to technology and potentially having access to devices 24 hours a day. More on this later in this chapter.

The meditation app Calm conducted a large study (2024) involving over 9000 adults aged 18–65 in the US and UK, and reported that there are generational differences when it comes to sleep. For example, Generation Z are 21 per cent more likely than Millennials to stay up at night, frequently or all the time. They're also 26 per cent more likely to be kept up at night by prolonged technology use compared to Millennials. Not great if you consider the previous advice in Chapter 9 regarding not going beyond an individual's sleep time if using a device pre-sleep (Bauducco *et al.*, 2024). Further, they reported that Generation Z and

Millennials have difficulty staying asleep, but 40 per cent of Generation Z struggle to fall asleep on more than half of the days in a week, which is 21 per cent higher than Millennials. Worryingly, only 35 per cent of Generation Z sleep more than seven hours a night, compared to 30 per cent of Millennials (Calm, 2024).

THE QUESTION OF SCREEN TIME

I discussed screen time in earlier chapters, but the explosion in technological devices within our homes over recent years, along with the recent Covid-19 pandemic, has resulted in a marked increase in the use of devices within the home, particularly by Generation Z, the individuals born into the digital revolution. They have never not known the internet and have grown up through a technology-savvy age. Consequently, screen time in this generation is higher than any previous generation and is, seemingly, influencing sleep, particularly if screen time is continued past normal bedtime (Bauducco *et al.*, 2024; Calm, 2024; Gradisar, personal communication). As lives become reduced to being held in a device that fits inside a coat pocket, its content accessible any time of day, sleep becomes ever more deprioritized to those unaware of its significance – a dangerous precedent to set for future generations. A good article in the UK newspaper *The Guardian* made an important point: 'we may be built to sleep, but the modern world isn't. Our schedules are tethered not to the sun but technology. We are awash in artificial light every hour, we feel that we can't afford to switch off' (Hunt, 2023).

The Catch-22 scenario of the benefits of remote working, online education resources and mobile entertainment devices means the decision about how to manage screen time is a challenging one. The advice in this book isn't about screen time and whether a person should engage with it or not, an emotive issue at the best of times. Simply, the information in this book is intended to provide an explanation of the potential impact of *bright light* exposure on sleep and why managing exposure to light at certain parts of the day is important for sleep. Chapter 9 covered this in more detail, but ultimately, attempting to avoid screens in a technological age is probably futile. One cannot ignore the fact that technology is here to stay. However, addressing the amount of exposure to screens that an individual has, particularly later in the day, is worth considering for overall sleep health. For technology use in the pre-sleep window, a 'harm minimization' approach is suggested. Activities such as putting any devices in the bedroom on flight mode, not using them later than the intended bedtime and using devices for less engaging activities, such as watching television instead of gaming, are recommended (Bauducco et al., 2024).

In addition, some individuals may be more susceptible than others to the adverse effects of technology on sleep. Therefore, any interventions should focus on their individual vulnerabilities. For example, individuals with low self-control might instead benefit from modifying their sleep environment so that it reduces temptation, by, for example, not keeping stimulating technology close to them in the bedroom. Conversely, some people may use technology in the bedroom to facilitate sleep, and removing all devices from the bedroom may not always be effective and potentially lead to more negative thoughts and cognitive arousal, and eventually fuel insomnia symptoms. Therefore, minimizing damage around sleep and technology should ideally be the focus when providing recommendations to clients, in addition to taking into consideration their age and familiarization with using devices pre-sleep (Bauducco et al., 2024).

Of course, sleep issues in relation to different generations and technology are not gender specific. However, if you consider that the current age of Generation Z is typically adolescents through to young adults, and the differences in sleep that appear once puberty begins, as described in Chapter 4, it is possible that Generation Z females have even more sleep-related challenges than previous generations.

FUTURE DIRECTIONS FOR HEALTH PROFESSIONALS AND SLEEP HEALTH EDUCATION

The good news is that sleep is becoming more and more of a conversation topic in public health and higher on the agenda of wellness leads in industry and education. The message about needing regular good sleep quality and quantity seems to be resonating more and more. Certainly, since I started my own consultancy focusing on sleep and recovery for performance, I have noticed an upsurge in interest around the topic of sleep health, with more demand from audiences from diverse spheres for sleep education workshops, webinars and information resources.

This demand for sleep knowledge also extends to a variety of sleep topics, such as shift work, sleep aids and female health (particularly popular), highlighting that people and employers are considering their sleep in more depth than ever before. An understanding of sleep is also championed through the fact that, within industry, employers are encouraged to provide fatigue-management systems for shift workers and educate employees about sleep health in general. The objective of most companies who request my input is to educate employees and employers about the overall health benefits of valuing, prioritizing and protecting your sleep (Espie, 2022a). Thank goodness for 'Wellbeing Wednesday' in the learning and development sphere!

Undoubtably, there is more awareness now of the impact of poor sleep on all aspects of human behaviour and society. Public knowledge is improving around the fact that sleep is behaviour driven, to a certain extent by a person's genetics, their attitudes and beliefs, and socially through, for example, their environment or stage of life. Having the awareness that sleep restriction will impact on a person's ability to thrive in daily life, to be safe, fully aware, have good relationships and be physically and mentally 'well' can therefore change a person's approach to sleep and create a cascade of lifelong, positive health effects. The hope is that if people can start to manage their sleep health better, then this will have a consequential positive effect on public health in the long term.

I know from my background supporting athletes in high-performance sport that more attention is now placed on sleep as part of the management of athletes' training and competition programmes. As mentioned previously, the traditional sports assign more emphasis these days to performance-enhancing behaviour, such as obtaining sufficient sleep. For those readers working with athletes, there is a flow diagram depicting a process for practitioners to help optimize and manage sleep for athletes in the 2021 Expert Consensus on Sleep and Athletes (Walsh *et al.*, 2021). This is a useful resource for those considering best courses of action in supporting athletes in their sleep health.

Outside of elite sport, a recent manifesto launched by the Sleep Charity (2024) brought to national attention the problem of sleep as a public health concern. In their report, the Sleep Charity described a *triple sleep deficit* to describe the public health crisis that the UK is experiencing in relation to sleep. First, they described a 'sleep stealing' environment, where sleep is underappreciated and misunderstood. The study conducted for the manifesto reported that 75 per cent of people in work said workplace stresses caused them sleep issues in the last six months, and one in three people were experiencing 'sleep poverty', where poor living conditions, noise pollution and uncomfortable sleep environments reduced their sleep quality. Alarmingly, just one in 20 people were aware of the links between poor sleep and serious health problems, such as cancer, stroke and obesity, and more than a third were unaware of best-practice sleep advice.

Second, the manifesto stated that there is a normalization of poor sleep within British society. Staggeringly, the study found that 69 per cent of people with sleep issues had yet to seek support from a health-care professional and have instead lived with their problem for an average of more than six years. Worryingly, only one in six people with insomnia symptoms had been diagnosed. The ramification of this is that, nationally, millions of people may be suffering in silence with a sleep disorder that could be seriously impacting their mental and physical health. As described previously in this chapter, this also has consequences for people engaging in 'high-risk' behaviours such as driving or operating machinery whilst sleepy. There is also the effect of sleep restriction on the individual, particularly in terms of their mood, with the propensity for a rise in aggression and violent behaviours being reported in the study.

Finally, the manifesto stated that there is a 'postcode lottery' when it comes to accessing the recommended first-line treatments for sleep disorders such as insomnia or sleep apnoea, the two leading sleep disorders in the UK. Additionally, some GPs lack knowledge of the treatments that exist for sleep disorders and, consequently, how to access them. For example, NICE recommends cognitive behavioural therapy for insomnia (CBT-I) as the first-line treatment for both short- and long-term insomnia. Whilst digital CBT-I is now more readily available, face-to-face CBT-I isn't, with few NHS Trusts offering both face-to-face and digital CBT-I. Equally, not all GPs are aware of the availability of this line of treatment or its success in treating insomnia.

Solutions to these problems are outlined in the manifesto and suggest changes at government level as being one of the most impactful solutions. If the UK government can take on board the message about a public health crisis in the UK in relation to sleep, then this will be an important move forward in creating change. Without a doubt, including sleep in existing public health campaigns, using sleep as a critical message in creating new public health campaigns and encouraging the knowledge development of GPs around sleep disorders and treatment pathways, in addition to making referral pathways more widely available for treatments such as CBT-I, will help health professionals take a monumental step towards improving the sleep of the nation.

TRAINING SLEEP PRACTITIONERS

To support some of the solutions proposed in the manifesto, training avenues for sleep practitioners need to be made available and existing pathways more accessible. Historically, guidance and education to become knowledgeable and skilled in sleep health education have been varied. If you are not a clinical professional or working in a sleep research domain, then there has, until recently, been little quality-assured accreditation for sleep practitioners in the UK.

The lack of personnel with specific knowledge of sleep would be helped by neophyte practitioners in healthcare professions (clinical and non-clinical), fitness and wider industries being trained from undergraduate (or equivalent) level onwards in the technicalities of sleep health. An increased emphasis on the physiology of sleep and its effects on a person's health in medical and allied health professionals' undergraduate degree courses would involve a seismic change in practice across the established health sciences and medical academia. I mentioned in Chapter 1 how little emphasis was placed on the topic of sleep in the health profession's academic courses. However, knowing the objective and subjective methods available to monitor sleep, potential treatment pathways and solutions for sleep issues would greatly enhance system-wide knowledge and understanding of sleep. One challenge to this is that the curriculum for health courses is already very full, so what would have to be modified in the current curriculum to allow space and time for better practitioner sleep education? This is a perpetual argument, but it is a change that could be impactful in terms of practitioner knowledge and improvements in public health by preventing the health consequences of poor sleep.

Fortunately, in addition to clinical and academic paths of study, the Sleep Charity have recently developed a range of sleep education courses suitable for professionals from health, social care, education, voluntary and the commercial sectors. They offer training courses through their Sleep Well Academy, which is an established and highly recommended provider of sleep training courses for professionals and families. Through the courses on offer, the Sleep Charity are unlocking the opportunities for people to train in sleep health education.

Other courses include the Oxford University-based Sleep and Circadian Neuroscience Institute Cognitive Behavioural Therapy for Insomnia Masterclass, a two-day masterclass for clinical professionals, including psychologists, psychiatrists, physicians, technologists, nurses, allied health professionals and clinical researchers. I have taken this course and found it incredibly useful in understanding the breadth of intervention options available through CBT-I, which has helped in explaining this method to those whom I educate about sleep health.

There is also the Edinburgh Sleep Medicine Course, which is a five-day course covering topics ranging from the basics of sleep science to learning how to set up your own sleep laboratory. The course is suitable for all health professionals with an interest in sleep medicine and is accredited by the Royal College of Physicians.

The Society of Behavioural Sleep Medicine also offer support in advancing the scientific approach to studying behavioural, psychological and physiological dimensions of sleep and sleep disorders, and application of this knowledge to improve the sleep of individuals and societies worldwide. Their mission is to set standards and promote excellence in behavioural sleep medicine healthcare, education and research. They have an index of behavioural sleep medicine practitioners worldwide (including CBT-I); details are provided in the resources section at the end of this book.

Other resources exist on the Sleep Charity's website to help support clients with sleep issues. They have various eBooks, a Teen Sleep Hub, podcasts and advice pages for a whole manner of aspects of sleep. Equally, the Sleep Foundation, based in America, have an extensive website full of resources and information about sleep. The British Sleep Society also have some useful information, but more allied to clinicians than healthcare professionals in general. They also offer regular webinars on topics related to sleep medicine for all members, and details can be found on their website (signposted at the end of the book).

Outside of the UK, you will need to research accredited sleep practitioners, and it's probably worth doing your homework before sending a client to a sleep practitioner, either in or outside the UK. As ever, if there is a clinical intervention required, then clients should be referred to the appropriate healthcare professional in the first instance, typically their GP.

SUMMARY

I hope this book has enabled you to understand sleep health in more detail and the impact it can have across a woman's lifespan. From puberty to fertility and pregnancy, postpartum, the menopause transition, and as caregivers and employees, women's sleep is affected.

I hope you now have some tools to help you brush up on your sleep health knowledge and enable you to have a dialogue around it in consultations with your clients. Please remember to reinforce with them that you cannot force sleep, but you can increase its likelihood. If they give themselves the opportunity to sleep and follow strategies to help it happen, then often sleep will improve as required (in a healthy adult without a sleep or circadian rhythm disorder).

The strategies provided in this book are intended as practical interventions to try if your clients experience poor sleep. If you suspect a person has a sleep or circadian rhythm disorder, then appropriate referral will be necessary, and signposts are available at the end of the book.

> This book is not going to solve the global problem of poor sleep, but if it goes some way towards helping support your clients who experience poor sleep, or spread education around sleep health, then it will have had a positive impact on someone's sleep.

From my early observations of sleep science literature, it certainly lacked detail around some of the nuances of female sleep and how we apply that knowledge. However, the science has developed, and women can now access information about their sleep for different phases of their lifespan. Therefore, raising awareness of and helping women understand their sleep health and how it might change or be affected throughout their lifespan is part of the solution to helping women sleep better. Nevertheless, there remains an awful lot more to understand in relation to women's sleep, in particular some of the more mechanistic reasons why and how sleep impacts on key phases in a woman's life or vice versa.

In writing this book, I often thought of what I needed when I was a practitioner supporting elite athletes and coaches and forging my understanding of sleep. Yes, there were sleep resources out there, but nothing that really spoke to me as a non-clinical practitioner focusing on supporting athletes, particularly female athletes, to try to improve, via good sleep health, their ability to consistently perform well in training and competition. I hope this book would fill that gap, if I could have that time again.

Finally, people often ask how I sleep. I don't want to be so arrogant as to assume this is particularly interesting to the reader, but it is a common query that I get asked. I don't mind reporting that, overall, I sleep very well. I am conscious of my practices around my sleep health and cognizant of the core values around good sleep health (i.e. prioritize, protect, value, personalize a sleep window and trust in sleep being a natural process that will happen), with a healthy dose of pragmatism too. I regularly get outdoors – having a young family helps with this – and I am grateful that I can fit in some kind of physical activity several times a week. At the time of writing, the perimenopause is rearing its head, so I accept that, at times, my sleep will be compromised in the same way as if there is an unexpected temporary life stress, or a social event that means a later night and time to bed. Overall, I give myself the opportunity to get good sleep on a regular basis and recognize the benefits that that gives me in terms of wellness and enjoyment in my daily life. I don't always get it right, and life can get in the way, but generally I am happy with my sleep. I hope this book allows you to be that too and also helps others you support. With that, I will end on a quote from the late Dr Allan Rechtschaffen, who was a seminal researcher in the study of the function of sleep:

> *If sleep does not serve an absolutely vital function, then it is the biggest mistake the evolutionary process has ever made. (Mignot, 2008)*

I like this quote as it is a reminder that sleep is not something invented by us humans or a product of the last 200 years' industrialization. It is a natural process, serving many biological functions to ultimately sustain life. So happy sleeping and enjoy the discovery of what works for you and your clients to get regular healthy sleep.

Resources

BOOKS

Chokroverty, S. & Ferini-Strambi, L. (eds) (2017). *Oxford Textbook of Sleep Disorders*. Oxford: Oxford University Press.

Keay, N. (2022). *Hormones, Health and Human Potential*. Keighley: Sequoia Books.

Logan, G. (2024). *The Midpoint Plan: Taking Charge of Your Health, Habits and Happiness to Thrive in Midlife and Beyond*. London: Little, Brown Book Group.

Leschziner, G. (ed.) (2022). *Oxford Handbook of Sleep Medicine*. Oxford: Oxford University Press.

Leschziner, G. (2022). *The Man Who Tasted Words: Inside the Strange and Startling World of Our Senses*. London: Simon & Schuster.

Smith, S. (2022). *The Story of the Cardiff and Vale Perinatal Mental Health Team January 1998–July 2020*. Surbiton: Grosvenor House Publishing.

ORGANIZATIONS

Action on Postpartum Psychosis

www.app-network.org

Active Pregnancy Foundation

www.activepregnancyfoundation.org

Active Women's Clinic

https://theactivewomensclinic.com

American Academy of Sleep Medicine

https://aasm.org

Alcohol Change UK

https://alcoholchange.org.uk

Anxiety UK

www.anxietyuk.org.uk

Association for Post-Natal Illness

https://apni.org

Barnardo's

www.barnardos.org.uk

Best Beginnings
Provides information about many aspects of pregnancy and parenting, including mental wellbeing, in the form of short video clips. Also provides a 'Baby Buddy' app to guide you through your pregnancy.

www.bestbeginnings.org.uk

Better Sleep Clinic

www.thebettersleepclinic.co.uk

Beyond Blue

www.beyondblue.org.au

British Association for Behavioural and Cognitive Psychotherapies
Lead organization for CBT in the UK and Ireland, where you can find details of all officially accredited CBT therapists.

www.babcp.com

British Dietetic Association

www.bda.uk.com

British Menopause Society

https://thebms.org.uk

British Nutrition Foundation

www.nutrition.org.uk

THE ESSENTIAL GUIDE TO WOMEN'S SLEEP

British Sleep Society

www.sleepsociety.org.uk

British Snoring and Sleep Apnoea Association

www.britishsnoring.shop

Bed Advice UK

Provides professional, unbiased and generic advice on everything consumers need to know about beds and mattresses to help with bed-buying.

https://bedadvice.co.uk

Calm

An app for guided meditation and sleep stories

www.calm.com

CPAP

A free public information resource for those seeking to learn more about sleep apnoea and snoring, and for those who are existing sleep apnoea patients on CPAP therapy.

www.cpap.co.uk

Daisy Network

For premature menopause.

www.daisynetwork.org

Doctor Care Anywhere

https://doctorcareanywhere.com

Endometriosis UK

www.endometriosis-uk.org

Gilchrist Performance

www.gilchristperformance.co.uk

GenM

https://gen-m.com

Global Dro

www.globaldro.com

Good Sleep Clinic

https://goodsleep.clinic

Health & Care Professions Council (HCPC)
A register of dietitians and other health professionals.

http://www.hcpc-uk.org

Healthtalk
A website using research to help people to feel better prepared, better informed and less alone in health matters.

www.healthtalk.org

Hope2Sleep
A registered charity run by sleep apnoea sufferers, CPAP and non-invasive ventilator users and sleep professionals – all of whom are passionate and committed to supporting people to get the safe restful sleep they deserve.

www.hope2sleep.co.uk

Maternal OCD
Support and information for women with perinatal obsessive compulsive disorder. X/Twitter support group: #Bumpsandmumsocdhr.

https://maternalocd.org

Informed Sport

www.informedsport.com

Menopause Café

www.menopausecafe.net

Menopause Matters

www.menopausematters.co.uk

Mental Health First Aid England

https://mhfaengland.org

Mind

Mind.org.uk

The Menopause Charity

www.themenopausecharity.org

My Menopause Centre

www.mymenopausecentre.com

National Bed Federation (NBF)

The recognized trade association representing UK manufacturers of beds and their suppliers.

www.bedfed.org.uk

Netmums

www.netmums.com

PANDAS Foundation UK

https://pandasfoundation.org.uk/what-is-pnd/perinatal-mental-health

PND and Me
Website and online support group for sufferers of perinatal mental illness with links to information and a range of resources around this topic. Set up by a mum who had postnatal depression. Includes peer support through X (formerly Twitter): #PNDHour & #PNDChat.

pndandme.co.uk

RAND
A research organization focusing on providing solutions to public policy challenges.

www.rand.org

Royal College of General Practitioners

www.rcgp.org.uk

Royal College of Psychiatrists

www.rcpsych.ac.uk

Royal Society of Medicine

www.rsm.ac.uk

Royal Society for the Prevention of Accidents (RoSPA)

www.rospa.com

The Sleep Charity

www.thesleepcharity.org.uk

The Sleep Foundation

www.sleepfoundation.org

Sleep Well Academy
The Sleep Charity's provider of sleep training courses for professionals and families.

https://sleepwellacademy.org.uk

Society of Behavioural Sleep Medicine

www.behavioralsleep.org

UK Anti-Doping

www.ukad.org.uk

Verity
UK PCOS charity

www.verity-pcos.org.uk

Women's Health Concern

www.womens-health-concern.org

World Anti-Doping Agency

www.wada-ama.org/en

World Sleep Society

https://worldsleepsociety.org

YoungMinds

www.youngminds.org.uk

Zarach
A charity committed to helping children and families who are living in poverty crisis.

https://zarach.org

TRAINING
The Sleep Charity: Foundation Sleep Workshop
Introductory course

https://sleepwellacademy.org.uk/course/foundation-sleep-workshop

The Sleep Charity: Sleep Success Workshop
With bolt-on for special educational needs and disabilities

https://sleepwellacademy.org.uk/course/sleep-success-workshop

The Sleep Charity: Sleep Tight Workshop
Supports practitioners with setting up and running their own sleep services with an evidence-based behavioural approach

https://sleepwellacademy.org.uk/course/sleep-tight-workshop

The Sleep Charity: Sleep Champion Workshop
Aimed at professionals working in secondary schools

https://sleepwellacademy.org.uk/course/sleep-champion-workshop

The Sleep Charity: Sleep Practitioner Course

https://sleepwellacademy.org.uk/course/sleep-practitioner-course

The Sleep Charity: Adult Sleep Training

https://sleepwellacademy.org.uk/course/adult-sleep-training

The Sleep Charity: Cognitive Behavioural Therapy for Insomnia

https://sleepwellacademy.org.uk/course/cognitive-behavioural-therapy-for-insomnia-cbt-i

The Sleep Charity: Workplace Sleep Ambassador Course

https://sleepwellacademy.org.uk/course/workplace-sleep-ambassador-course

Oxford University Sleep and Circadian Neuroscience Institute
Cognitive Behavioural Therapy for Insomnia Masterclass (2 days)

www.scni.ox.ac.uk/study-with-us/oxford-online-programme-in-sleep-medicine/cognitive-behavioural-therapy-for-insomnia

Edinburgh Sleep Medicine Course (5 days)

www.sleepconsultancyltd.co.uk/courses/edinburgh-sleep-medicine

OTHER RESOURCES
Beating Bipolar
Programme aiming to improve understanding of bipolar. Includes a module about pregnancy for women with bipolar: https://ibpf.org/resource/bipolar-online-support-group-for-perinatal-pregnancy-and-postpartum-moms-birthing-people

https://ibpf.org/resource/beating-bipolar

Best Use of Medicines in Pregnancy (BUMPS)

www.medicinesinpregnancy.org

British Snoring and Sleep Apnoea Association: STOPBang questionnaire

https://britishsnoring.co.uk/stop_bang_questionnaire.php

Epworth Sleepiness Scale

https://epworthsleepinessscale.com/about-the-ess

Health and Safety Executive: Managing shift work: Health and safety guidance

www.hse.gov.uk/pubns/books/hsg256.htm

Mental Health Foundation: Sleep and mental health

www.mentalhealth.org.uk/explore-mental-health/a-z-topics/sleep-and-mental-health

NHS: *A Guide to Your CPAP*

www.england.nhs.uk/wp-content/uploads/2023/11/A-guide-to-your-CPAP-easy-read.pdf

NHS: Endometriosis

www.nhs.uk/conditions/endometriosis

NHS: Insomnia

www.nhs.uk/conditions/insomnia

NHS: Menopause

www.nhs.uk/conditions/menopause

NHS: Polycystic ovary syndrome

www.nhs.uk/conditions/polycystic-ovary-syndrome-pcos

NHS: Obstructive sleep apnoea

www.nhs.uk/conditions/sleep-apnoea

Professor Jason Ellis: *Coping with Stress Related Sleep Loss* leaflet
Available by contacting Jason Ellis at:

www.northumbria.ac.uk/about-us/our-staff/e/jason-ellis

The Fawcett Society: Menopause and the Workplace Report

www.fawcettsociety.org.uk/menopauseandtheworkplace

Royal College of Psychiatrists: What are Perinatal Mental Health Services?

www.rcpsych.ac.uk/mental-health/treatments-and-wellbeing/what-are-perinatal-mental-health-services

The Sleep Charity: Podcast

https://thesleepcharity.org.uk/information-support/podcast

The Sleep Charity: Sleep diary

https://thesleepcharity.org.uk/information-support/adults/sleep-diary

The Sleep Charity: Sleep poverty

https://thesleepcharity.org.uk/get-involved/sleep-poverty

The Sleep Charity: Teen Sleep Hub – Teens and Young People

https://teensleephub.org.uk/teens-young-people

The Sleep Charity: Useful Resources, including World of Sleep eBook

https://thesleepcharity.org.uk/information-support/useful-resources

The Sleep Foundation: What Is Orthosomnia?

www.sleepfoundation.org/orthosomnia

The Sleep Foundation: Caffeine and Sleep

www.sleepfoundation.org/nutrition/caffeine-and-sleep

The Sleep Foundation: Alcohol and Sleep

www.sleepfoundation.org/nutrition/alcohol-and-sleep

The Sleep Foundation: Is 7 hours of sleep enough?

www.sleepfoundation.org/sleep-faqs/is-7-hours-of-sleep-enough

The Sleep Foundation: Women & Sleep

www.sleepfoundation.org/women-sleep

Sleepio: A free programme using CBT-I to treat insomnia

www.sleepio.com

Tommy's
Mental health before, during and after pregnancy

www.tommys.org/pregnancy-information/im-pregnant/mental-wellbeing/mental-health-during-and-after-pregnancy

UK Anti-Doping: Athlete Support Personnel

www.ukad.org.uk/athlete-support-personnel

References

Aggeler, M. (2024, 12 September). Eating too much and working in bed: Experts share 10 worst sleep mistakes. *The Guardian Australia*. www.theguardian.com/wellness/article/2024/sep/11/top-10-sleep-mistakes-experts

de Alcantara Borba, D., Reis, R. S., de Melo Lima, P. H. T., Facundo, L. A. *et al*. (2020). How many days are needed for a reliable assessment by the Sleep Diary? *Sleep Science*, 13(1), 49–53.

Alimoradi, Z., Gozal, D., Tsang, H. W. H., Lin, C. Y. *et al*. (2022). Gender-specific estimates of sleep problems during the COVID-19 pandemic: Systematic review and meta-analysis. *Journal of Sleep Research*, 31(1), 1–16

Alnawwar, M. A., Alraddadi, M. I., Algethmi, R. A., Salem, G. A., Salem, M. A. & Alharbi, A. A. (2023). The effect of physical activity on sleep quality and sleep disorder: A systematic review. *Cureus*, 15(8), e43595.

American Academy of Sleep Medicine (2023). International Classification of Sleep Disorders – Third Edition, Text Revision Summary of Diagnostic Criteria Changes. https://aasm.org/clinical-resources/international-classification-sleep-disorders

American Academy of Sleep Medicine and Sleep Research Society (2015). Recommended amount of sleep for a healthy adult: A joint consensus statement of the American Academy of Sleep Medicine and Sleep Research Society. *Sleep*, 8(6), 843–844.

Andersen, M. L., Araujo, P., Frange, C. & Tufik, S. (2018). Sleep disturbance and pain: A tale of two common problems. *Chest*, 154(5), 1249–1259.

Auger, N., Healy-Profitós, J. & Wei, S. Q. (2021). In the arms of Morpheus: Meta-analysis of sleep and fertility. *Fertility and Sterility*, 115(3), 596–598.

Baattaiah, B. A., Alharbi, M. D., Babteen, N. M., Al-Maqbool, H. M., Babgi, F. A. & Albatati, A. A. (2023). The relationship between fatigue, sleep quality, resilience, and the risk of postpartum depression: An emphasis on maternal mental health. *BMC Psychology*, 11(10), 1–17.

Bacaro, V., Chiabudini, M., Buonanno, C., De Bartolo, P. *et al*. (2020. Insomnia in the Italian population during Covid-19 outbreak: A snapshot on one major risk factor for depression and anxiety. *Frontiers in Psychiatry*, 11, 579107.

Baek, J. B. (2023). Menstrual disturbances and its association with sleep disturbances: A systematic review. *BMC Women's Health*, 23, 470–489

Baglioni, C., Espie, C. A., Spiegelhalder, K., Gavriloff, D. & Riemann, D. (2022). Recommendation of the European Academy for Cognitive-Behavioural Therapy for Insomnia (CBT-I) for High Quality Training for Health Professionals. In C. Baglioni, C. A. Espie & D. Reimann (eds) *Cognitive-Behavioural Therapy for Insomnia (CBT-I) Across the Life Span: Guidelines and Clinical Protocols for Health Professionals* (pp. 243–250). Hoboken, NJ: Wiley Blackwell.

Baker, F. C. & Driver, H. S. (2007). Circadian rhythms, sleep, and the menstrual cycle. *Sleep Medicine*, 8(6), 613–622.

Banks, S. & Dinges, D. F. (2007). Behavioural and physiological consequences of sleep restriction. *Journal of Clinical Sleep Medicine*, 3(5), 519–528.

Banno, M., Harada, Y., Taniguchi, M., Tobita, R. *et al.* (2018). Exercise can improve sleep quality: A systematic review and meta-analysis. *PeerJ*, 11(6), e5172.

Barnes, S. (2022). Travelgate: Sleep and the WNBA's working conditions. Engaging Sports. https://thesocietypages.org/engagingsports/2022/09/15/travelgate-sleep-and-the-wnbas-working-conditions

Baron, K. G., Abbott, S., Jao, N., Manalo, N. & Mullen, R. (2017). Orthosomnia: Are some patients taking the quantified self too far? *Journal of Clinical Sleep Medicine*, 13(2), 351–354.

Bauducco, S., Pillion, M., Bartel, K., Reynolds, C., Kahn, M. & Gradisar, M. A. (2024). Bidirectional model of sleep and technology use: A theoretical review of how much, for whom, and which mechanisms. *Sleep Medicine Reviews*. doi: 10.1016/j.smrv.2024.101933

Bazeley, A., Marren, C. & Shepherd, A. (2022). *Menopause and the Workplace.* Fawcett Society. www.fawcettsociety.org.uk/Handlers/Download.ashx?IDMF=9672cf45-5f13-4b69-8882-1e5e643ac8a6

BBC News (2023, 24 January). 'Menopause leave' trial rejected by ministers. www.bbc.co.uk/news/uk-politics-64381216

Bed Advice UK (2024). Fire Safety in the Bedroom this Autumn. https://bedadvice.co.uk/fire-safety-in-the-bedroom-this-autumn

Beecham, A. (2022). The surprisingly scientific reason why Bear Grylls wants you to start calling your alarm clock an 'opportunity clock'. Stylist. www.stylist.co.uk/health/sleep/bear-grylls-alarm-clock-waking-up-easier/738871

Beroukhim, G., Esencan, E. & Seifer, D. B. (2022). Impact of sleep patterns upon female neuroendocrinology and reproductive outcomes: A comprehensive review. *Reproductive Biology and Endocrinology*, 20(16), 1–17.

Besedovsky, L., Lange, T. & Born, J. (2012). Sleep and immune function. *European Journal of Physiology*, 463, 121–137.

Bestbier, L. & Williams, T. (2017). The immediate effects of deep pressure on young people with autism and severe intellectual difficulties: A case series demonstrating individual differences. *Occupational Therapy International*. doi: 10.1155/2017/7534972

Bjornsdottir, E., Thorarinsdottir, E. H., Lindberg, E., Benediktsdottir, B. *et al.* (2024). Association between physical activity over a 10-year period and current insomnia symptoms, sleep duration and daytime sleepiness: A European population-based study. *British Medical Journal Open*, 14(3), 1–10.

Boege, H. L., Bhatti, M. Z. & St-Onge, M. P. (2021). Circadian rhythms and meal timing: Impact on energy balance and body weight. *Current Opinion in Biotechnology*, 70, 1–6.

Bonde, J. P., Jørgensen, K. T., Bonzini, M. & Palmer, K. T. (2012). Miscarriage and occupational activity: A systematic review and meta-analysis regarding shift work, working hours, lifting, standing, and physical workload. *Scandinavian Journal of Work Environment Health*, 39(4), 325–334.

Bonnar, D., Bartel, K., Kakoschke, N. & Lang, C. (2018). Sleep interventions designed to improve athletic performance and recovery: A systematic review of current approaches. *Sports Medicine*, 48, 683–703.

Bonnar, D., Lee, S., Gradisar, M. & Suh, A. (2019). Risk factors and sleep intervention considerations in esports: A review and practical guide. *Sleep Medicine Research*, 10, 59–66.

Borbély, A. A. (1982). A two process model of sleep regulation. *Human Neurobiology*, 1(3), 195–204.

Borbély, A. A., Daan, S., Wirz-Justice, A. & Deboer, T. (2016). The two-process model of sleep regulation: A reappraisal. *Journal of Sleep Research*, 25, 131–143.

Bowling, G (2023). Not just a women's problem. Improving menopause workplace policy and support. Nuffield Health. www.nuffieldhealth.com/article/breaking-the-stigma-the-biggest-workplace-menopause-challenges-and-how-to-tackle-them

Breathe Diagnostics (2020). Wake Up to the Dangers of Sleep Apnea! https://breathediagnostics.com/sleep-apnea-101

Brewis, J., Beck, V., Davies, A. & Metheson, J. (2017). *Menopause Transition: Effects on Women's Economic Participation.* Department for Education. www.gov.uk/government/publications/menopause-transition-effects-on-womens-economic-participation

British Dietetics Association (2023). Fluid (Water and Drinks) and Hydration. www.bda.uk.com/resource/fluid-water-drinks.html

Brooke-Wavell, K., Skelton, D, A., Barker, K, L., Clark, E. M. *et al.* (2022). Strong, steady and straight: UK consensus statement on physical activity and exercise for osteoporosis. *British Journal of Sports Medicine*, 56(15), 837–846.

Broomfield, N., Espie, C., MacMahon, K., Macphee, L. & Taylor, L. (2006). The attention-intention-effort pathway in the development of psychophysiologic insomnia: A theoretical review. *Sleep Medicine Reviews*, 10, 215–245.

Brown, A. M. & Gervais, N. J. (2020). Role of ovarian hormones in the modulation of sleep in females across the adult lifespan. *Endocrinology, 161*(9), bqaa128.

Brown, A. M. & Gervais, N. J. (2022). Corrigendum to: 'Role of ovarian hormones in the modulation of sleep in females across the adult lifespan'. *Endocrinology*, 163(1), bqab227.

Bryan, L. & Peters, B. (2024). Periodic limb movement disorder: What it is, what it feels like, its possible causes, and how it's addressed. Sleep Foundation. www.sleepfoundation.org/periodic-limb-movement-disorder

Bryan, L. & Singh, A. (2024). Alcohol and sleep. Sleep Foundation. www.sleepfoundation.org/nutrition/alcohol-and-sleep

Burke, T. M., Lisman, P. J., Maguire, K., Skeiky, L. *et al.* (2020). Examination of sleep and injury among college football athletes. *Journal of Strength and Conditioning Research*, 34(3), 609–616.

Buysse, D. J., Reynolds III, C. F., Monk, T. H., Berman, S. R. & Kupfer, D. J. (1989). The Pittsburgh Sleep Quality Index: A new instrument for psychiatric practice and research. *Journal of Psychiatric Research*, 28(2), 193–213.

Byrne, P. (2017). The trouble with sleep watches [blog post]. Byrne Fatigue Consulting. http://byrne-co.com/the-trouble-with-sleep-watches

Caetano, G., Bozinovic, I., Dupont, C., Léger, D., Lévy, R. & Sermondade, N. (2021). Impact of sleep on female and male reproductive functions: A systematic review. *Fertility and Sterility*, 115(3), 715–731.

Cai, C., Vandermeer, B., Khurana, R., Nerenberg, K. *et al.* (2019). The impact of occupational shift work and working hours during pregnancy on health outcomes: A systematic review and meta-analysis. *American Journal of Obstetrics and Gynaecology*, 221(6), 563–576.

Calm (2024). Calm presents *The Snooze Report*: A study on sleep in the US and UK. www.calm.com/blog/the-snooze-report

Cappadona, R., De Giorgi, A., Di Simone, E., Zucchi, B. *et al.* (2021). Sleep, dreams, nightmares, and sex-related differences: A narrative review. *European Review for Medical and Pharmacological Sciences*, 25(7), 3054–3065.

Chauhan, G. & Tadi, P. (2022). Physiology, Postpartum Changes. StatPearls. Treasure Island, FL: StatPearls Publishing. www.statpearls.com/point-of-care/27550

Chennaoui, M., Bougard, C., Drogou, C., Langrume, C. *et al.* (2016). Stress biomarkers, mood states, and sleep during a major competition: 'Success' and 'failure' athlete's profile of high-level swimmers. *Frontiers in Physiology*, 7, 94.

Chennaoui, M., Pierrick, J. A., Sauvet, F. & Leger, D. (2015). Sleep and exercise: A reciprocal issue? *Sleep Medicine Reviews*, 20, 59–72.

Cheon, J. & Kim, M. (2022). Comprehensive effects of various nutrients on sleep. *Sleep and Biological Rhythms*, 20, 449–458.

Cherpak, C. E. & Van Lare, S. J. (2019). Menstrual cycle fluctuations of progesterone and the effect on sleep regulation. *Journal of Restorative Medicine*, 8, 1–15.

Cho, M. K. (2015). Thyroid dysfunction and subfertility. *Clinical Experiments in Reproductive Medicine*, 42(4), 131–135.

Chung, S. A., Wolf, T. K. & Shapiro, C. M. (2009). Sleep and health consequences of shift work in women. *Journal of Women's Health*, 18(7), 965–977.

Clawson, B. C., Durkin, J. & Aton, S. J. (2016). Form and function of sleep spindles across the lifespan. *Neural Plasticity*, 14, 1–16.

Comtet, H., Geoffroy, P. A., Kobayashi Frisk, M., Hubbard, J. *et al.* (2019). Light therapy with boxes or glasses to counteract effects of acute sleep deprivation. *Scientific Reports*, 9(1), 18073.

Cooper, A. & Mullen, l. (2023). *No Crib for a Bed: The Impact of the Cost-of-Living Crisis on Bed Poverty*. Barnardo's. www.barnardos.org.uk/sites/default/files/2023-09/report-no-crib-bed-poverty-cost-living-crisis.pdf

Copeland, B. (2024). Artificial intelligence. *Encyclopedia Britannica*. www.britannica.com/technology/artificial-intelligence

Dillner, L. (2017, 9 October). Is it healthier to sleep naked rather than in pyjamas? *The Guardian*. www.theguardian.com/lifeandstyle/2017/oct/09/is-it-healthier-to-sleep-naked-rather-than-in-pyjamas-fertility

Dinges, D. F. (1992). Adult Napping and Its Effects on Ability to Function. In C. Stampi (ed.) *Why We Nap* (pp. 118–134). Boston, MA: Birkhäuser.

Dinges, D. F. (2014). The growth of sleep science and the role of sleep. *Sleep*, 37(1), 7–8.

Dolezal, B. A., Neufeld, E. V., Boland, D. M., Martin, J. L. & Cooper, C. B. (2017). Interrelationship between sleep and exercise: A systematic review. *Advances in Preventive Medicine*. doi: 10.1155/2017/1364387.

Dorsey, A., De Lecea, L. & Jennings, K. J. (2021). Neurobiological and hormonal mechanisms regulating women's sleep. *Frontiers in Neuroscience*, 14, 625397.

Driver, H. S. and Taylor, S. R. (2000). Exercise and sleep. *Sleep Medicine Review*, 4(4), 387–402.

Duffy, J. F. & Czeisler, C. A. (2009). Effect of light on human circadian physiology. *Sleep Medicine Clinics*, 4(2), 165–177.

Duvet Advisor (n.d.). TOGs Explained. www.duvetadvisor.co.uk/home-page/togs-explained

Ekblom, O., Nyberg, G., Bak, E. E., Ekelund, U. & Marcus, C. (2012). Validity and comparability of a wrist-worn accelerometer in children. *Journal of Physical Activity and Health*, 9(3), 389–393.

Elliott-Sale, K. J., Minahan, C. L., de Jonge, X. A. J., Ackerman, K. E. *et al.* (2021). Methodological considerations for studies in sport and exercise science with women as participants: A working guide for standards of practice for research on women. *Sports Medicine*, 51(5), 843–861.

Erten Uyumaz, B., Feijs, L. & Hu, J. (2021). A review of digital cognitive behavioural therapy for insomnia (CBT-I apps): Are they designed for engagement? *International Journal Environmental Research for Public Health*, 18(6), 2929.

Espie, C. A. (2012). *Overcoming Insomnia and Sleep Problems: A Self-Help Guide Using Cognitive Behavioral Techniques*. London: Little, Brown Book Group.

Espie, C. A. (2022a). The '5 principles' of good sleep health. *Journal of Sleep Research*, 31(3), 1–7.

Espie, C. A. (2022b). The importance of sleep at each stage of life. Psychology Today. www.psychologytoday.com/gb/blog/the-big-sleep/202210/the-importance-sleep-each-stage-life

Fabbri, M., Alessia, B., Martoni, M., Meneo, D., Tonetti, L. & Natale, V. (2021). Measuring subjective sleep quality: A review. *International Journal of Environmental Research and Public Health*, 18(3), 1082.

Falkingham, J. C., Evandrou, M., Qin, M. & Vlachantoni, A. (2022). Prospective longitudinal study of 'Sleepless in Lockdown': Unpacking differences in sleep loss during the coronavirus pandemic in the UK. *British Medical Journal Open*, 12(1), 1–18.

Fatemeh, G., Sajjad, M., Niloufar, R., Neda, S., Leila, S. & Khadijeh, M. (2022). Effect of melatonin supplementation on sleep quality: A systematic review and meta-analysis of randomized controlled trials. *Journal of Neurology*. doi: 10.1007/s00415-020-10381-w.

The Fawcett Society (2022). *Menopause and the Workplace*. www.fawcettsociety.org.uk/Handlers/Download.ashx?IDMF=9672cf45-5f13-4b69-8882-1e5e643ac8a6

Finan, P. H., Goodin, B. R. & Smith, M. T. (2013). The association of sleep and pain: An update and a path forward. *Journal of Pain*, 14(12), 1539–1552.

Fonseca, A. P. L. M., de Azevedo, C. V. M. & Santos, R. M. R. (2021). Sleep and health-related physical fitness in children and adolescents: A systematic review. *Sleep Science*, 14(4), 357–365.

Francis-Devine, B. & Hutton, G. (2024). *Women and the UK Economy*. UK Parliament. https://commonslibrary.parliament.uk/research-briefings/sn06838

Frank, M. G. & Benington, J. H. (2006). The role of sleep in memory consolidation and brain plasticity: Dream or reality? *Neuroscientist*, 12(6), 477–488.

Franklin, K. A., Sahlin, C., Stenlund, H. & Lindberg, E. (2013). Sleep apnoea is a common occurrence in females. *European Respiratory Journal*, 41(3), 610–615.

Freeman, D., Sheaves, B., Goodwin, G. M., Yu, L. M. *et al.* (2021). Sleep and health-related physical fitness in children and adolescents: A systematic review. *Sleep Science*, 14(4), 357–365.

Fryer, B. (2006, October). Sleep deficit: The performance killer. *Harvard Business Review*. https://hbr.org/2006/10/sleep-deficit-the-performance-killer

Fullagar, H. K., Skorski, S., Duffield, R., Hammes, D., Coutts, A. J. & Meyer, T. (2015). Sleep and athletic performance: The effects of sleep loss on exercise performance, and physiological and cognitive responses to exercise. *Sports Medicine*, 45(2), 161–186.

Gandhi, A. V., Mosser, E. A., Oikonomou, G. & Prober, D. A. (2015). Melatonin is required for the circadian regulation of sleep. *Neuron*, 85, 1193–1199.

Garcia, L. S. (2020). Melatonin and its effects: The truth behind this popular supplement. Semantic Scholar. www.semanticscholar.org/paper/Problems-in-assessment-of-acute-melatonin-overdose.-Holliman-Chyka/0fed5b6ee5ac7887e4e375375257a58942c7426b

Gardiner, C., Weakley, J., Burke, L. M., Roach, G. D. *et al.* (2023). The effect of caffeine on subsequent sleep: A systematic review and meta-analysis. *Sleep Medicine Reviews*, 69, 101764.

Gavriloff, D. (2024). Insomnia [webinar]. British Sleep Society, April.

GenM (2020). *Generation Menopause: Invisibility Report*. https://gen-m.com/wp-content/uploads/2021/09/GenM-Invisibility-Report.pdf

Gleeson, M. & Pyne, D. B. (2016). Respiratory inflammation and infections in high-performance athletes. *Immunology and Cell Biology*, 94(2), 124–131.

Goldberg, M., Pairot de Fontenay, B., Blache, Y. & Debarnot, U. (2024). Effects of morning and evening physical exercise on subjective and objective sleep quality: An ecological study. *Journal of Sleep Research*, 33(1), e13996.

Goldstein, C. A. and Smith, Y. A. (2016). Sleep, circadian rhythms and fertility. *Current Sleep Medicine Reports*, 2, 206–217.

Gorvett, Z. (2022). The forgotten medieval habit of 'two sleeps'. BBC Future. www.bbc.com/future/article/20220107-the-lost-medieval-habit-of-biphasic-sleep

Gottesmann, C. (2002). GABA mechanisms and sleep. *Neuroscience*, 111(2), 231–239.

Gradisar, M. (2024). *Sleep Cycle* [podcast]. https://podcasts.apple.com/us/podcast/sleep-and-technology/id1696621991

Grandner, M. (2022). Basics of sleep physiology and behaviour [webinar]. University of Arizona Sleep Webinar series. www.sleephealthresearch.com/archive_essentials_bsm.html

Grandner, M. A., Hale, L., Moore, M. & Patel, N. P. (2010a). Mortality associated with short sleep duration: The evidence, the possible mechanisms, and the future. *Sleep Medicine Review*, 14(3), 191–203.

Grandner, M. A., Patel, N. P., Gehrman, P. R., Perlis, M. L. & Pack, A. I. (2010b). Problems associated with short sleep: Bridging the gap between laboratory and epidemiological studies. *Sleep Medicine Review*, 14(4), 239–247.

Grier, T., Dinkeloo, E., Reynolds, M. & Jones, B. H. (2020). Sleep duration and musculoskeletal injury incidence in physically active men and women: A study of US Army Special Operation Forces soldiers. *Sleep Health*, 6(3), 344–349.

The Guardian (2011). the Great British Sleep Survey. www.theguardian.com/lifeandstyle/gallery/2011/jan/29/great-british-sleep-survey

Gupta, L., Morgan, K. & Gilchrist, S. (2016). Does elite sport degrade sleep quality? A systematic review. *Sports Medicine*, 47(7), 1–17.

Gupta, L., Morgan, K., North, C. & Gilchrist, S. (2021). Napping in high-performance athletes: Sleepiness or sleepability? *European Journal of Sport Science*, 21(3), 321–330.

Gupta, S., Bansal, K. & Saxena, P. (2022). A clinical trial to compare the effects of aerobic training and resistance training on sleep quality and quality of life in older adults with sleep disturbance. *Sleep Science*, 15(2), 188–195.

Gurubhagavatula, I., Barger, L. K., Barnes, C. M., Basner, M. *et al.* (2021). Guiding principles for determining work shift duration and addressing the effects of work shift duration on performance, safety, and health: Guidance from the American Academy of Sleep Medicine and the Sleep Research Society. *Journal of Clinical Sleep Medicine*, 17(11), 2283–2306.

Haack, M., Simpson, N., Sethna, N., Kaur, S. & Mullington, J. (2020). Sleep deficiency and chronic pain: Potential underlying mechanisms and clinical implications. *Neuropsychopharmacology*, 45, 205–216.

Hafner, M., Stepanek, M., Taylor, J., Troxel, W. M. & Van Stolk, C. (2017). Why sleep matters – the economic costs of insufficient sleep: A cross-country comparative analysis. *Rand Health Quarterly*, 6(4), 11.

Halson, S. L. (2008). Nutrition, sleep and recovery. *European Journal of Sport Science*, 8(2), 119–126.

Halson, S. L. (2014). Sleep in elite athletes and nutritional interventions to enhance sleep. *Sports Medicine*, 44(1), S13–S23.

Halson, S. L., Burke, L. M. & Pearce, J. (2019). Nutrition for travel: From jet lag to catering. *International Journal of Sport Nutrition and Exercise Metabolism*, 29(2), 228–235.

Harrington, J. (2001). Health effects of shift work and extended hours of work. *Occupational and Environmental Medicine*, 58, 68–72.

Hatcher, K. M., Smith, R. L., Chiang, C., Li, Z., Flaws, J. A. & Mahoney, M. M. (2020). Association of phthalate exposure and endogenous hormones with self-reported sleep disruptions: Results from the Midlife Women's Health Study. *Menopause*, 27(11), 1251–1264.

Haufe, A. & Leeners, B. (2023). Sleep disturbances across a woman's lifespan: What is the role of reproductive hormones? *Journal of Endocrine Society*, 7, 1–14.

Hauri, P. J. (1977). *The Sleep Disorders (Current Concepts)*. Kalamazoo, MI: Upjohn.

Health and Safety Executive (2002). *The Track Obstruction by a Road Vehicle and Subsequent Train Collisions at Great Heck 28 February 2001*. www.railwaysarchive.co.uk/documents/HSE_HeckRep001.pdf

Henpicked (2021). Menopause at work: Employers' legal responsibilities now. https://menopauseintheworkplace.co.uk/articles/menopause-at-work-employers-legal-responsibilities-now

Herxheimer, A. & Petrie, K. J. (2002). Melatonin for the prevention and treatment of jet lag. *Cochrane Database of Systematic Reviews*, 2002(2). doi: 10.1002/14651858.CD001520.

Hill, K. (1996). The demography of menopause. *Maturitas*, 23(2), 113–127.

Hoang, H. T. X., Yeung, W. F., Truong, Q. T. M., Le, C. T. *et al.* (2024). Sleep quality among non-hospitalized COVID-19 survivors: A national cross-sectional study. *Frontiers in Public Health*, 11, 1281012.

Holzman, D. C. (2010) What's in a color? The unique human health effects of blue light. *Environmental Health Perspectives*, 118(1), A22–A27.

Horne, J. A. & Ostberg, O. (1976). A self-assessment questionnaire to determine morningness-eveningness in human circadian rhythms. *International Journal of Chronobiology*, 4(2), 97–110.

Houses of Parliament Committee (2021). *Written evidence from Menopause Self Care (MSC) CIC [MEW0041]*. https://committees.parliament.uk/writtenevidence/39156/html

Houses of Parliament: Parliamentary Office of Science and Technology (2018). *Shift Work, Sleep and Health*. https://researchbriefings.files.parliament.uk/documents/POST-PN-0586/POST-PN-0586.pdf

Huang, K. & Ihm, J. (2021). Sleep and injury risk. *Current Sports Medicine Reports*, 20(6), 286–290.

Hunt, E. (2023, 5 January). Take more breaks at work, put your head in the freezer...an expert's eight simple tips for better sleep. *The Guardian*. www.theguardian.com/lifeandstyle/2023/jan/05/take-more-breaks-at-work-put-your-head-in-the-freezer-an-experts-eight-simple-tips-for-better-sleep

Hyyppa, M. T. & Kronholm, E. (1989). Quality of sleep and chronic illnesses. *Journal of Clinical Epidemiology*, 42(7), 633–638.

Informed Health (2006). Heavy Periods. www.informedhealth.org/heavy-periods.html

International Menopause Society (2024). Mission and Vision of the IMS. www.imsociety.org/about-us/mission/?v=7885444af42e

Jackson, P., Holmes, A., Hilditch, C., Reed, N., Smith, L. & Merat, N. (2011). *Fatigue and Road Safety: An Evidence-Based Review. Research Report*. London: Department for Transport.

Jehan, S., Auguste, E., Hussain, M., Pandi-Perumal, S. R. *et al*. (2016). Sleep and premenstrual syndrome. *Journal of Sleep Medicine Disorders*, 3(5), 1061.

Jein, G. (2020). *Sleeping with David Baddiel. Episode 6: A Sleep-Friendly Society*. [audiobook]. www.audible.co.uk/podcast/Ep-6-A-Sleep-Friendly-Society/B08GC6815W

Johns, M. W. (1990). A new method for measuring daytime sleepiness: The Epworth Sleepiness Scale. *Sleep*, 14(6), 540–545.

Johnston, I. (2017, 2 January). 'Catastrophic' lack of sleep in modern society is killing us, warns leading sleep scientist. *The independent*. www.independent.co.uk/news/sleep-deprivation-epidemic-health-effects-tired-heart-disease-stroke-dementia-cancer-a7964156.html

Kalmbach, D. A., Buysse, D. J., Cheng, P., Roth, T., Yang, A. & Drake, C. L. (2020). Nocturnal cognitive arousal is associated with objective sleep disturbance and indicators of physiologic hyperarousal in good sleepers and individuals with insomnia disorder. *Sleep Medicine*, 71, 151–160.

Keay, N. (2022). *Hormones, Health and Human Potential*. Keighley: Sequoia Books.

Kelley, P., Lockley, S. W., Foster, R. G. & Kelley, J. (2015). Synchronizing education to adolescent biology: 'Let teens sleep, start school later'. *Learning, Media and Technology*, 40(2), 210–226.

Khoury, J. & Doghramji, K. (2015). Primary sleep disorders. *Psychiatric Clinics of North America*, 38(4), 683–704.

Kirshenbaum, J. S., Coury, S. M., Colich, N. L., Manber, R. & Gotlib, I. H. (2023). Objective and subjective sleep health in adolescence: Associations with puberty and affect. *Journal of sleep research*, 32(3).

Kline, C. (2014). The bidirectional relationship between exercise and sleep: Implications for exercise adherence and sleep improvement. *American Journal of Lifestyle Medicine*, 8(6), 375–379.

Kline, C. (2020). Sleep Quality. In M. D. Gellman (ed.) *Encyclopedia of Behavioural Medicine* (pp. 1811–1813). Cham, Switzerland: Springer International Publishing.

Kloss, J. D., Perlis, M. L., Zamzow, J. A., Culnan, E. J. & Gracia, C. R. (2015). Sleep, sleep disturbance, and fertility in women. *Sleep Medicine Reviews*, 22, 78–87.

Kräuchi, K., Fattori, E., Giordano, A., Falbo, M. *et al*. (2018). Sleep on a high heat capacity mattress increases conductive body heat loss and slow wave sleep. *Physiology and Behaviour*, 1(185), 23–30.

Kredlow, M. A., Capozzoli, M. C., Hearon, B. A., Calkins, A. W. & Otto, M. W. (2015). The effects of physical activity on sleep: A meta-analytic review. *Journal of Behavioural Medicine*, 38, 427–449.

Krystal, A. D., Edinger, J., Wohlgemuth, W. & Marsh, G. R. (1998). Sleep in peri-menopausal and post-menopausal women. *Sleep Medicine Reviews*, 2(4), 243–253.

Kushida, C. A., Chang, A., Gadkary, C., Guilleminault, C., Carrillo, O. & Dement, W. C. (2001). Comparison of actigraphic, polysomnographic and subjective assessment of sleep parameters in sleep-disordered patients. *Sleep Medicine*, 2(5), 389–396.

Lambiase, M. J., Gabriel, K. P., Chang, Y. F., Kuller, L. H. & Matthews, K. A. (2014). Utility of Actiwatch sleep monitor to assess waking movement behaviour in older women. *Medicine and Science in Sports and Exercise*, 46(12), 2301–2307.

Lapin, B. R., Bena, J. F., Walia, H. K. & Moul, D. E. (2018). The Epworth Sleepiness Scale: Validation of one-dimensional factor structure in a large clinical sample. *Journal of Clinical Sleep Medicine*, 14(8), 1293–1301.

Lateef, O. M. & Akintubosun, M. O. (2020). Sleep and reproductive health. *Journal of Circadian Rhythms*, 18(1), 1–11.

Lee, S., Bonnar, D., Roane, B., Gradisar, M. *et al*. (2021). Sleep characteristics and mood of professional esports athletes: A multi-national study. *International Journal of Environmental Research and Public Health*, 14, 18(2), 664.

Leeder, J., Glaister, M., Pizzoferro, K., Dawson, J. & Pedlar, C. (2012). Sleep duration and quality in elite athletes measured using wristwatch actigraphy. *Journal of Sports Sciences*, 30(6), 541–545.

Leger, D., Elbaz, M., Raffray, T., Metlaine, V. B. & Duforez, F. (2008). Sleep management and the performance of eight sailors in the Tour de France a la voile yacht race. *Journal of Sports Sciences*, 26(1), 21–28.

Leschziner, G. (ed.) (2020). *The Secret World of Sleep: Journeys Through the Nocturnal Mind*. London: Simon & Schuster.

Leschziner, G. (ed.) (2022a). *Oxford Handbook of Sleep Medicine*. Oxford Medical Handbooks. Online edn. Oxford: Oxford Academic.

Leschziner, G. (2022b). *The Man Who Tasted Words: Inside the Strange and Startling World of Our Senses*. London: Simon & Schuster.

Levy, A. (2022). Insomnia is a $5 billion business – and this former sleep doctor thinks it's time for a new approach. CNBC. www.cnbc.com/2022/12/23/insomnia-former-sleep-doctor-promotes-treating-it-as-a-phobia.html

Lewis, B. A., Gjerdingen, D., Schuver, K., Avery, M. & Marcus, B. H. (2018). The effect of sleep pattern changes on postpartum depressive symptoms. *BMC Women's Health*. doi:10.1186/s12905-017-0496-6

Li, J., Vitiello, M. V. & Gooneratne, N. S. (2022). Sleep in normal aging. *Sleep Medicine Clinics*, 17(2), 161–171.

Lufkin, B. (2021, 25 January). The coronasomnia phenomenon keeping you from getting sleep. BBC Worklife. www.bbc.com/worklife/article/20210121-the-coronasomnia-phenomenon-keeping-us-from-getting-sleep

MacLean, J. E., Fitzgerald, D. A. & Waters, K. A. (2015). Developmental changes in sleep and breathing across infancy and childhood. *Paediatric Respiratory Reviews*, 16(4), 276–284.

Mah, C. D., Mah, K. E., Kezirian, E. J. & Dement, W. C. (2011). The effects of sleep extension on the athletic performance of collegiate basketball players. *Sleep*, 34(7), 943–950.

Mellow, M. L., Crozier, A. J., Dumuid, D., Wade, A. T. *et al.* (2022). How are combinations of physical activity, sedentary behaviour and sleep related to cognitive function in older adults? A systematic review. *Experimental Gerontology*. doi: 10.1016/j.exger.2022.111698.

Menopause Mandate (2024). *Menopause Mandate Survey 2024: The Results*. www.menopausemandate.com/mm24-survey-results

Mental Health First Aid England (2023). Mental Health First Aiders. https://mhfaengland.org/organisations/workplace/mental-health-first-aid

Mental Health Foundation (2020). Taking Sleep Seriously: Sleep and our Mental Health. www.mentalhealth.org.uk/explore-mental-health/publications/taking-sleep-seriously

Mignot, E. (2008). Why we sleep: The temporal organization of recovery. *PLoS Biology*, 6(4), e106.

Mihaila, S. (2023). UK design company to launch AI menopause management app. Femtech World. www.femtechworld.co.uk/news/uk-design-company-to-launch-ai-menopause-management-app

Miller, D. J., Sargent, C., Roach, G. D., Scanlan, A. T., Vincent, G. E. & Lastella, M. (2020). Moderate-intensity exercise performed in the evening does not impair sleep in healthy males. *European Journal of Sport Science*, 20(1), 80–89.

Milner, C. E. & Cote, K. A. (2009). Benefits of napping in healthy adults: Impact of nap length, time of day, age and experience with napping. *Journal of Sleep Research*, 18, 272–281.

Mindell, J. A., Bartle, A., Abd Wahab, N., Ahn, Y. *et al.* (2011). Sleep education in medical school curriculum: A glimpse across countries. *Sleep Medicine*, 12(9), 928–931.

Mitler, M. M., Carskadon, M. A., Czeisler, C. A., Dement, W. C., Dinges, D. F. & Graeber, R. C. (1988). Catastrophes, sleep, and public policy: Consensus report. *Sleep*, 11(1), 100–109.

Moe, K. E. (2004). Hot flashes and sleep in women. *Sleep Medicine Reviews*, 8(6), 487–497.

Money and Mental Health Policy Institute (2022). Cost of living squeeze could cause national mental health crisis – with 11m UK adults saying they feel 'unable to cope' due to rising costs. www.moneyandmentalhealth.org/press-release/cost-of-living-crisis

Moore, I. S., Crossley, K. M., Bo, K., Mountjoy, M. *et al.* (2023). Female athlete health domains: A supplement to the International Olympic Committee consensus statement on methods for recording and reporting epidemiological data on injury and illness in sport. *British Journal of Sports Medicine*, 57(18), 1164–1174.

Morgan, K. (2016). Presentation. Sleep to Win workshop, English Institute of Sport, March.

Morin, C. M. & Carrier, J. (2021). The acute effects of the COVID-19 pandemic on insomnia and psychological symptoms. *Sleep Medicine*, 77, 346–347.

Moser, D., Anderer, P., Gruber, G., Parapatics, S. *et al.* (2008). Sleep classification according to AASM and Rechtschaffen & Kales: Effects on sleep scoring parameters. *Sleep* 32(2), 139–149.

Mountjoy, M., Sundgot-Borgen, J., Burke, L., Ackerman, K. E. *et al.* (2018). International Olympic Committee (IOC) consensus statement on relative energy deficiency in sport (RED-S): 2018 update. *International Journal of Sport Nutrition and Exercise Metabolism*, 28(4), 316–331.

Murphy, P. J. & Campbell, S. S. (2007). Sex hormones, sleep, and core body temperature in older postmenopausal women. *Sleep*, 30(12), 1788–1794.

Mycroft, L. (2022). Why FE needs radical rest. FE News. www.fenews.co.uk/exclusive/why-fe-needs-radical-rest

Mycroft, L. (2023). What we've learned about Radical Rest. FE News. www.fenews.co.uk/exclusive/what-weve-learned-about-radical-rest

Myllymäki, T., Kyrolainen, H., Savolainen, K., Hokka, L. *et al.* (2011). Effects of vigorous late-night exercise on sleep quality and cardiac autonomic activity. *Journal of Sleep Research*, 20, 146–153.

Nagata, C., Shimizu, H., Takami, R., Hayashi, M., Takeda, N. & Yasuda, K. (1999). Hot flushes and other menopausal symptoms in relation to soy product intake in Japanese women. *Climacteric*, 2(1), 6–12.

National Bed Federation (2020). How Much Does A Good Bed Cost? https://bedadvice.co.uk/how-much-does-a-good-bed-cost

Netzer, N. C., Eliasson, A. H. & Strohl, K. P. (2003). Women with sleep apnoea have lower levels of sex hormones. *Sleep and Breathing*, 7(1), 25–29.

Neurolaunch (2024). Sleep improvement after quitting alcohol: A timeline of recovery. https://neurolaunch.com/when-does-sleep-improve-after-quitting-alcohol

NHS (2022a). Endometriosis. www.nhs.uk/conditions/endometriosis

NHS (2023). Severe vomiting in pregnancy. www.nhs.uk/pregnancy/related-conditions/complications/severe-vomiting

NHS (2024). Dealing with Stress. www.nhs.uk/every-mind-matters/mental-health-issues/stress

NICE (2021). *Continuous Positive Airway Pressure for the Treatment of Obstructive Sleep Apnoea/Hypopnoea Syndrome*. NICE Guideline TA139. www.nice.org.uk/guidance/ta139/resources/continuous-positive-airway-pressure-for-the-treatment-of-obstructive-sleep-apnoeahypopnoea-syndrome-pdf-82598202209221

NICE (2024). *Menopause: Identification and Management*. NICE Guideline NG23. www.nice.org.uk/guidance/ng23

Nogueira, H. A., de Castro, C. T., da Silva, D. C. G. & Pereira, M. (2023). Melatonin for sleep disorders in people with autism: Systematic review and meta-analysis. *Progress in Neuro-Psychopharmacology and Biological Psychiatry*, 123, 110695.

Nowakowski, S. (2021). Sleep and Menopause: It's a hot mess! [webinar]. University of Arizona Sleep Webinar series. www.sleephealthresearch.com/archive_essentials_bsm.html

Nowakowski, S., Meers, J. & Heimbach, E. (2013). Sleep and women's health. *Sleep Medicine Research*, 4(1), 1–22.

Nuffield Health (2023). Major new survey highlights impact of cost-of-living crisis on mental and physical wellbeing. www.nuffieldhealth.com/article/the-healthier-nation-index-release#sleep

Nunes, F. R., Ferreira, J. M. & Bahamondes, L. (2015). Pain threshold and sleep quality in women with endometriosis. *European Journal of Pain*, 19(1), 15–20.

Nunn, C. L., Samson, D. R. & Krystal, A. D. (2016). Shining evolutionary light on human sleep and sleep disorders. *Evolutionary Medicine in Public Health*, 3(1), 227–243.

Oda, S. & Shirakawa, K. (2014). Sleep onset is disrupted following pre-sleep exercise that causes large physiological excitement at bedtime. *European Journal of Applied Physiology*, 114(9), 1789–1799.

Office for National Statistics (2021). Birth Characteristics in England and Wales: 2021. www. ons.gov.uk/peoplepopulationandcommunity/birthsdeathsandmarriages/livebirths/ bulletins/birthcharacteristicsinenglandandwales/2021

Ohayon, M., Wickwire, E. M., Hirshkowitz, M., Albert, S. M. *et al.* (2017). National Sleep Foundation's sleep quality recommendations: First report. *Sleep Health*, 3(1), 6–19.

Ong, J. L., Golkashani, H. A., Ghorbani, S., Wong, K. F. *et al.* (2024). Selecting a sleep tracker from EEG-based, iteratively improved, low-cost multisensor, and actigraphy-only devices. *Sleep Health*, 10(1), 9–23.

Pacheco, D. (2023). How bedroom temperatures and bedding choices impact your sleep. Sleep Foundation. www.sleepfoundation.org/sleep-news/bedroom-tempera tures-and-bedding-choices-affect-sleep

Pacheco, D. & Callender, E. (2024). Women & Sleep. Sleep Foundation. www.sleepfoundation. org/women-sleep

Pacheco, D. & Cotliar, D. (2024). Caffeine and Sleep. Sleep Foundation. www.sleepfoundation. org/nutrition/caffeine-and-sleep

Pacheco, D. & Rehman, A. (2023). Pain and Sleep. Sleep Foundation. www.sleepfoundation. org/physical-health/pain-and-sleep

Pacheco, D. & Wells, A. (2024). Restless Leg Syndrome (RLS): What it is, its causes and symptoms, and how it can be addressed to improve sleep. Sleep Foundation. www. sleepfoundation.org/restless-legs-syndrome

PANDAS Foundation UK (2024). Perinatal Mental Health. https://pandasfoundation.org. uk/what-is-pnd/perinatal-mental-health

Pankhurst, F. P. & Home, J. A. (1994). The influence of bed partners on movement during sleep. *Sleep*, 17(4), 308–315.

Papadopoulos, D. & Etindele Sosso, F. A. (2023). Socioeconomic status and sleep health: A narrative synthesis of 3 decades of empirical research. *Journal of Clinical Sleep Medicine*, 19(3), 605–620.

Park, D., Kim, S., Shin, C. & Suh, S. (2021). Prevalence of and factors associated with night-mares in the elderly in a population based cohort study. *Sleep Medicine*, 78, 15–23.

Park, S. Y., Oh, M. K., Lee, B. S., Kim, H. G. *et al.*, (2015). The effects of alcohol on quality of sleep. *Korean Journal of Family Medicine*, 36(6), 294–299.

De Pasquale, C., El Kazzi, M., Sutherland, K., Shriane, A. E. *et al.* (2024). Sleep hygiene – What do we mean? A bibliographic review. *Sleep Medicine Reviews*. doi: 10.1016/j. smrv.2024.101930.

Pengo, M. F., Won, C. H. & Bourjeily, G. (2018). Sleep in women across the life span. *Chest*, 154(1), 196–206.

Pereira, N., Naufel, M. F., Ribeiro, E. B., Tufik, S. & Hachul, H. (2020). Influence of dietary sources of melatonin on sleep quality: A review. *Journal of Food Science*, 85(1), 5–13.

Piéron, H. (1913). *Le problème physiologique du sommeil* [The physiological problem of sleep]. Paris: Masson.

Poussel, M., Laroppe, J., Hurdiel, R., Girard, J. *et al.* (2015). Sleep management strategy and performance in an extreme mountain ultra-marathon. *Research in Sports Medicine*, 23(3), 330–336.

Psychreg (2024). BACP urges UK governments to address mental health crisis worsened by cost of living pressures. www.psychreg.org/bacp-urges-uk-governments-address-mental-health-crisis-worsened-cost-living-pressures

Purtill, J. (2024). Sleep-tracking devices are wiring the world for the study of sleep. What will we find? ABC News. www.abc.net.au/news/science/2024-09-24/sleep-tracking-wearables-making-whole-world-sleep-lab/104300328

Qiu, J. & Morales-Muñoz, I. (2022). Associations between sleep and mental health in ado-lescents: Results from the UK Millennium Cohort Study. *International Journal Environ-mental Research and Public Health*, 19(3), 1868.

Ramar, K., Malhotra, R. K., Carden, K. A., Martin, J. L. *et al.* (2021). Sleep is essential to health: American Academy of Sleep position statement. *Journal of Clinical Sleep Medicine*, 17, 2115–2119.

Rausch-Phung, E. & Singh, A. (2023). Is 7 Hours of Sleep Enough? Sleep Foundation. www.sleepfoundation.org/sleep-faqs/is-7-hours-of-sleep-enough

Rechtschaffen, A. & Kales, A. (eds) (1968). *A Manual of Standardized Terminology, Techniques and Scoring System for Sleep Stages of Human Subjects*. Los Angeles, CA: Brain Information Service, Brain Research Institute.

Reid, K. J., Kräuchi, K., Grimaldi, D., Sbarboro, J. *et al.* (2021). Effects of manipulating body temperature on sleep in postmenopausal women. *Sleep Medicine*, 81, 109–115.

Reilly, T. & Edwards, B. (2007). Altered sleep–wake cycles and physical performance in athletes. *Physiology and Behaviour*, 90(2–3), 274–284.

Riemann, D., Espie, C. A., Altena, E., Arnardottir, E. S. *et al.* (2023). The European Insomnia Guideline: An update on the diagnosis and treatment of insomnia 2023. *Journal of Sleep Research*, 32(6), e14035.

Reimers, K. (2019). *The Clinician's Guide to Geriatric Forensic Evaluations*. London: Academic Press.

Robotham, D. (2011). Sleep as a public health concern: Insomnia and mental health. *Journal of Public Mental Health*, 10(4), 234–237.

Romiszewski, S., May, F. E. K., Homan, E. J., Norris, B., Miller, M. A. & Zeman, A. (2020). Medical student education in sleep and its disorders is still meagre 20 years on: A cross-sectional survey of UK undergraduate medical education. *Journal of Sleep Research*. doi: 10.1111/jsr.12980.

Rouhi, S., Topcu, J., Egorova-Brumley, N. & Jordan, A. S. (2023). The impact of sleep disturbance on pain perception: A systematic review examining the moderating effect of sex and age. *Sleep Medicine Reviews*. doi: 10.1016/j.smrv.2023.101835.

Royal Society for the Prevention of Accidents (2024). *Road Safety Factsheet: Driver Fatigue and Road Collisions*. www.rospa.com/getmedia/25999a67-6e67-4a8c-b32d-13b5c1090010/Driver-Fatigue-Factsheet-2022-updated.pdf

Rugvedh, P., Gundreddy, P. & Wandile, B. (2023). The menstrual cycle's influence on sleep duration and cardiovascular health: A comprehensive review. *Cureus*, 15(10), e47292.

Sadeh, A. (2011). The role and validity of actigraphy in sleep medicine an update. *Sleep Medicine Review*, 15(4), 259–267.

Sadeh, A. & Acebo, C. (2002). The role of actigraphy in sleep medicine. *Sleep Medicine Reviews*, 6(2), 113–124.

Samuels, C. H. (2008). Sleep, recovery, and performance: The new frontier in high-performance athletics. *Neurologic Clinics*, 26, 169–180.

Samuels, C. H., James, L., Lawson, D. & Meeuwisse, W. (2016). The Athlete Sleep Screening Questionnaire: A new tool for assessing and managing sleep in elite athletes. *British Journal of Sports Medicine*, 50, 418–422.

Saner, E. (2019, 17 June). Why sleep trackers could lead to the rise of insomnia – and orthosomnia. *The Guardian*. www.theguardian.com/lifeandstyle/2019/jun/17/why-sleeptrackers-could-lead-to-the-the-rise-of-insomnia-and-orthosomnia

Sargent, C., Lastella, M., Halson, S. L. & Roach, G. D. (2021). How much sleep does an elite athlete need? *International Journal of Sports Physiology and Performance*, 16(12), 1746–1757.

Scamardella, F., Russo, N. & Napolitano, F. (2020). The phenomenon of load management. *Journal of Physical Education and Sport*, 20, 2306–2309.

Schaedel, Z., Holloway, D., Bruce, D. & Rymer, J. (2021). Management of sleep disorders in the menopausal transition. *Post Reproductive Health*, 27(4), 209–214.

Schönauer, M. & Pöhlchen, D. (2018). Sleep spindles. *Current Biology*, 28(19), 1129–1130.

Schwartz, J. R. L. & Roth, T. (2008). Neurophysiology of sleep and wakefulness: Basic science and clinical implications. *Current Neuropharmacology*, 6, 367–378.

Scott, A. J., Webb, T. L., Martyn-St James, M., Rowse, G. & Weich, S. (2021). Improving sleep quality leads to better mental health: A meta-analysis of randomised controlled trials. *Sleep Medicine Reviews*, 60, 101556.

Shen, W. & Stearns, V. (2009). Treatment strategies for hot flushes. *Expert Opinion on Pharmacotherapy*, 10(7), 1133–1144.

Siddarth, D., Siddarth, P. & Lavretsky, H. (2014). An observational study of the health benefits of yoga or tai chi compared to aerobic exercise in community-dwelling middle-aged and older adults. *American Journal of Geriatric Psychiatry*, 22(3), 272–273.

Silva, A., Queiroz, S. S., Winckler, C., Vital, R. *et al.* (2012). Sleep quality evaluation, chronotype, sleepiness and anxiety of Paralympic Brazilian athletes: Beijing 2008 Paralympic Games. *British Journal of Sports Medicine*, 46(2), 150–154.

Silver, R. M., Hunter, S., Reddy, U. M., Facco, F. *et al.* (2019). Prospective evaluation of maternal sleep position through 30 weeks of gestation and adverse pregnancy outcomes. *Obstetrics and Gynecology*, 134(4), 667–676.

Skarpsno, E. S., Mork, P. J., Nilsen, T. I. L. & Holtermann, A. (2017). Sleep positions and nocturnal body movements based on free-living accelerometer recordings: Association with demographics, lifestyle, and insomnia symptoms. *Nature and Science of Sleep*, 1(9), 267–275.

The Sleep Charity (2023). *The National Sleep Helpline Impact Report September 2021–September 2023.*

The Sleep Charity (2024). Dreaming of Change: A Manifesto for Sleep. https://thesleepcharity.org.uk/get-involved/sleep-manifesto-2024

The Sleep Council (2017). *The Great British Bedtime Report.* www.sleep-hero.co.uk/the-great-british-bedtime-report

Spielman, A, J. (1986). Assessment of insomnia. *Clinical Psychology Review*, 6(1), 11–25.

Statuta, S. M., Asif, I. M. & Drezner, J. A. (2017). Relative energy deficiency in sport (RED-S). *British Journal of Sports Medicine*, 51, 1570–1571.

Steiger, A. (2003). Sleep and endocrinology. *Journal of International Medicine*, 254, 13–22.

Stocker, L. J., Macklon, N. S., Cheong, Y. C. & Bewley, S. J. (2014). Influence of shift work on early reproductive outcomes: A systematic review and meta-analysis. *Obstetrics and Gynecology*, 124(1), 99–110.

Sturdee, D. W. (2008). The menopausal hot flush – anything new? *Maturitas*, 60(1), 42–49.

Stutz, J., Eiholzer, R. & Spengler, C. M. (2019). Effects of evening exercise on sleep in healthy participants: A systematic review and meta-analysis. *Sports Medicine*, 49(2), 269–287.

Summer, J. & Rehman, A. (2022). What Is Orthosomnia? Sleep Foundation. www.sleepfoundation.org/orthosomnia

Svetieva, E., Clerkin, C. & Ruderman, M. N. (2017). Can't sleep, won't sleep: Exploring leaders' sleep patterns, problems, and attitudes. *Consulting Psychology Journal: Practice and Research*, 69(2), 80–97.

Takahashi, Y., Kipnis, D. M. & Daughaday, W. H. (1968). Growth hormone secretion during sleep. *Journal of Clinical Investigation*, 47, 2079–2090.

Tandon, V. R., Sharma, S., Mahajan, A., Mahajan, A. & Tandon, A. (2022). Menopause and sleep disorders. *Journal of Mid-Life Health*, 13(1), 26–33.

Thomas, K. A. & Burr, R. L. (2006). Melatonin level and pattern in postpartum versus nonpregnant nulliparous women. *Journal of Obstetric, Gynecologic and Neonatal Nursing*, 35(5), 608–615.

Thornton, H., Duthie, G. M., Pitchford, N., Delaney, J. A., Benton, D. T. & Dascombe, B. J. (2016). Effects of a 2-week high intensity training camp on sleep activity of professional rugby league athletes. *International Journal of Sports Physiology and Performance.* doi: 10.1123/ijspp.2016-0414

Thorpy, M. J. (2012). Classification of sleep disorders. *Neurotherapeutics*, 9(4), 687–701.

Thun, E., Bjorvatn, B., Flo, E., Harris, A. & Pallesen, S. (2015). Sleep, circadian rhythms, and athletic performance. *Sleep Medicine Reviews*, 23, 1–9.

Trades Union Congress (2018). Number of People Working Night Shifts up by More Than 150,000 in 5 Years. www.tuc.org.uk/news/number-people-working-night-shifts-more-150000-5-years

Tryon, W. W. (1996). Nocturnal activity and sleep assessment. *Clinical Psychology Review*, 16(3), 197–213.

UK Anti Doping (2023). Managing Supplement Risks. www.ukad.org.uk/athletes/managing-supplement-risks

UK Parliament (2022). Menopause and the Workplace. https://publications.parliament.uk/pa/cm5803/cmselect/cmwomeq/91/report.html

UK Parliament (2024). *House of Commons Women and Equalities Committee: Health Barriers for Girls and Women in Sport. Third Report of Session 2023–24.* https://committees.parliament.uk/publications/43602/documents/216689/default

Valipour, A., Lothaller, H., Rauscher, H., Zwick, H., Burghuber, O. C. & Lavie, P. (2007). Gender-related differences in symptoms of patients with suspected breathing disorders in sleep: A clinical population study using the sleep disorders questionnaire. *Sleep*, 30(3), 312–319.

Van Deun, D., Willemen, T., Verhaert, V., Haex, B., Van Huffel, S. & Vander Sloten, J. (2015). Ambient Intelligence in the Bedroom. In K. Curran (ed.) *Recent Advances in Ambient Intelligence and Context-Aware Computing* (pp. 122–142). Hershey, PA: IGI Global.

Vanderlinden, J., Boen, F. & van Uffelen, J. G. Z. (2020). Effects of physical activity programs on sleep outcomes in older adults: A systematic review. *International Journal of Behavioural Nutrition and Physical Activity*. doi:10.1186/s12966-020-0913-3.

Venter, R. E. (2012). Role of sleep in performance and recovery of athletes: A review article. *South African Journal for Research in Sport, Physical Education and Recreation*, 34(1), 167–184.

Vincent, K. & Tracey, I. (2008). Hormones and their interaction with the pain experience. *Reviews in Pain*, 2(2), 20–24.

Vivian-Taylor, J. & Hickey, M. (2014). Menopause and depression: Is there a link? *Maturitas*, 79(2), 142–156.

Voitsidis, P., Gliatas, I., Bairachtari, V., Papadopoulou, K. *et al.* Insomnia during the COVID-19 pandemic in a Greek population. *Psychiatry Research*, 289, 113076.

Walker, M. (2021). *What Is Sleep?* [podcast]. https://podcasts.apple.com/us/podcast/01-what-is-sleep/id1578319619?i=1000530723890

Walker, M. (2024a). *Sleep and Menopause* [podcast]. https://podcasts.apple.com/us/podcast/69-sleep-menopause/id1578319619?i=1000648736212

Walker, M. (2024b). *Ask Me Anything Part 9 – THC, Melatonin, and Defining 'Enough Sleep'* [podcast]. https://podcasts.apple.com/us/podcast/ask-me-anything-part-9-thc-melatonin-and-defining/id1578319619?i=1000664328121

Walker, M. (2024c). *Sleep and Relationships* [podcast]. https://podcasts.apple.com/us/podcast/78-sleep-relationships-with-dr-wendy-troxel/id1578319619?i=1000663656231

Wallop, H. (2014, 14 May). Are you getting enough sleep? *The Telegraph*. www.telegraph.co.uk/news/health/news/10827613/Are-you-getting-enough-sleep.html

Walsh, N. P., Halson, S. L., Sargent, C., Roach, G. D. *et al.* (2021). Sleep and the athlete: Narrative review and 2021 expert consensus recommendations. *British Journal of Sports Medicine*, 55(7), 356–368.

Wang, F. & Boros, S. (2021). The effect of physical activity on sleep quality: A systematic review. *European Journal of Physiotherapy*, 23(1), 11–18.

Wang, W. L., Chen, K. H., Pan, Y. C., Yang, S. N. & Chan, Y. Y. (2020). The effect of yoga on sleep quality and insomnia in women with sleep problems: A systematic review and meta-analysis. *BMC Psychiatry*, 20(1), 1–19.

Waterhouse, J., Reilly, T., Atkinson, G. & Edwards, B. (2007). Jet lag: Trends and coping strategies. *The Lancet*, 369(9567), 1117–1129.

Waterhouse, J., Reilly, T. & Edwards, B. (2004). The stress of travel. *Journal of Sports Sciences*, 22, 946–966.

Watson, A. M. (2017). Sleep and athletic performance. *Current Sports Medicine Reports*, 16(6), 413–418.

Watson, N. F., Badr, M. S., Belenky, G., Bliwise, D. L. *et al.* (2015). Recommended amount of sleep for a healthy adult: A joint consensus statement of the American Academy of Sleep Medicine and Sleep Research Society. *Journal of Clinical Sleep Medicine*, 11(6), 591–592.

Waxenbaum, J. A., Reddy, V. & Varacallo, M. (2023). Anatomy, Autonomic Nervous System. StatPearls. Treasure Island, FL: StatPearls Publishing. www.statpearls.com/point-of-care/32322

Weibel, J., Lin, Y. S., Landolt, H. P., Kistler, J. *et al.* (2021). The impact of daily caffeine intake on nighttime sleep in young adult men. *Scientific Reports*, 11, 4668.

Wickwire, E. M., Geiger-Brown, J., Scharf, S. M. & Drake, C. L. (2017). Shift work and shift work sleep disorder: Clinical and organizational perspectives. *Chest*, 151(5), 1156–1172.

Wilkinson, K. & Shapiro, C. (2013). Development and validation of the Nonrestorative Sleep Scale (NRSS). *Journal of Clinical Sleep Medicine*, 9(9), 929–937.

Wimms, A., Woehrle, H., Ketheeswaran, S., Ramanan, D. & Armitstead, J. (2016). Obstructive sleep apnoea in women: Specific issues and interventions. *Biomedical Research International*. doi: 10.1155/2016/1764837.

Winnebeck, E. (2024). Understanding Circadian Rhythms and Sleep [webinar]. Available at: BSS Webinars – BSS (sleepsociety.org.uk)

Wirz-Justice, A., Skene, D. J. and Münch, M. 2021. The relevance of daylight for humans. *Biochemical Pharmacology*, 191, 114304.

Woods, N. F. & Mitchell, E. S. (2010). Sleep symptoms during the menopausal transition and early post-menopause: Observations from the Seattle Midlife Women's Health Study. *Sleep*, 33(4), 539–549.

Woolroom (2024). *Clean Sleep Report*. www.thewoolroom.com/images/pdf/Clean-Sleep-Report-2024-Rebrand-digi.pdf

World Anti-Doping Agency (2021). *2021 World Anti-Doping Code 2021*. www.wada-ama.org/sites/default/files/resources/files/2021_wada_code.pdf

Xie, L., Kang, H., Xu, Q., Chen, M. J. *et al.* (2013). Sleep drives metabolite clearance from the adult brain. *Science*, 18(342), 1241–1224.

Xing, X., Xue, P., Li, S. X., Zhou, J. & Tang, X. (2020). Sleep disturbance is associated with an increased risk of menstrual problems in female Chinese university students. *Sleep and Breathing*, 24, 1719–1727.

Yang, P. Y., Ho, K. H., Chen, H. C. & Chien, M. Y. (2012). Exercise training improves sleep quality in middle-aged and older adults with sleep problems: A systematic review. *Journal of Physiotherapy*, 58(3), 157–163.

Yasuda, J., Kishi, N. & Fujita, S. (2023). Association between time from dinner to bedtime and sleep quality indices in the young Japanese population: A cross-sectional study. *Dietetics*, 2(2), 140–149.

Youngstedt, S. D. & Kline, C. E. (2006). Epidemiology of exercise and sleep. *Sleep and Biological Rhythms*, 4, 215–221.

de Zambotti, M., Colrain, I. M., Javitz, H. S. & Baker, F. C. (2014). Magnitude of the impact of hot flashes on sleep in perimenopausal women. *Fertility and Sterility*, 102(6), 1708–1715.

Zhao, J., Tian, Y., Nie, J., Xu, J. & Liu, D. (2012). Red light and the sleep quality and endurance performance of Chinese female basketball players. *Journal of Athletic Training*, 47(6), 673–678.

Zuraikat, F. M. & St-Onge, M. P. (2020). The Influence of Diet on Sleep. In R. R. Watson & V. R. Preedy (eds) *Neurological Modulation of Sleep* (pp. 205–215). London: Academic Press.

Zuraikat, F. M., Wood, R. A., Barragán, R. & St-Onge, M. P. (2021). Sleep and diet: Mounting evidence of a cyclical relationship. *Annual Review of Nutrition*, 41(1), 309–332.

Subject Index

Sub-headings in *italics* indicate tables and figures.

Author Index

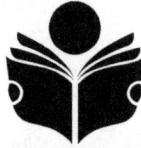

RAISING READERS
Books Build Bright Futures

Dear Reader,

We'd love your attention for one more page to tell you about the crisis in children's reading, and what we can all do.

Studies have shown that reading for fun is the **single biggest predictor of a child's future life chances** – more than family circumstance, parents' educational background or income. It improves academic results, mental health, wealth, communication skills, ambition and happiness.[1]

The number of children reading for fun is in rapid decline. Young people have a lot of competition for their time. In 2024, 1 in 10 children and young people in the UK aged 5 to 18 did not own a single book at home.[2]

Hachette works extensively with schools, libraries and literacy charities, but here are some ways we can all raise more readers:

- Reading to children for just 10 minutes a day makes a difference
- Don't give up if children aren't regular readers – there will be books for them!
- Visit bookshops and libraries to get recommendations
- Encourage them to listen to audiobooks
- Support school libraries
- Give books as gifts

There's a lot more information about how to encourage children to read on our website: **www.RaisingReaders.co.uk**

Thank you for reading.

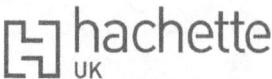

hachette
UK

1   National Literacy Trust, 'Book Ownership in 2024', November 2024, https://literacytrust.org.uk/research-services/research-reports/book-ownership-in-2024
2   OECD, '21st-Century Readers: Developing Literacy Skills in a Digital World', OECD Publishing, Paris, 2021, https://www.oecd.org/en/publications/21st-century-readers_a83d84cb-en.html